DEDICATION

This book is dedicated to my wonderful wife Ramona, who has amazing communication skills along with a powerful prophetic and intercessor anointing. It is truly humbling and scary living with such a powerhouse. She models and inspires me with her incredible life of purity, integrity and pursuit of Jesus. To my daughter Kimberly, a radical follower of Jesus who impacts the secular world as she interacts with people in a nonreligious and powerful way through her words and her life. To those who desire to invade the world with the kingdom of God through signs and wonders according to Mark 16:15-18. To every person who has a need to be healed of any disease or sickness. And to Jesus, my wonderful king, Lord and Savior, My Heavenly Father, and to Holy Spirit Who so patiently leads me in life.

FOREWARD

This work is the fourth and a major revision of what was originally called, "3 Days to Defeat Cancer." This revision has not only more than tripled the size of the original work, but the scope and material covered will prove invaluable to anyone who is seeking physical or emotional healing. The material covered is very comprehensive and relates to many issues we are faced with in life. Addressed are hindrances to physical healing, the role of forgiveness in healing, healing of heart wounds, practical keys to build faith, belief, a godly identity, and how to develop intimacy with the Lord.

In the Appendix are worksheets and prayers to overcome some common hindrances to physical healing as well as bringing healing to wounded hearts. Also included are life giving prayers, along with a daily healing declaration prayer.

INTRODUCTION

I don't believe there is anything more controversial than healing, especially when we speak about terminal diseases and conditions. Controversial or not, it's far better to face the issues, rather than ignore them. Ignoring health issues is tantamount to accepting defeat and being willing to live with a debilitating disease, or worse resigning yourself to an early death. Although it is true that the death rate is 100%, for everyone, the greater truth is that death does not have to be a result of a disease or sickness. I firmly believe that when it is time for our departure, we were meant to peacefully leave this world healthy, and not die from sickness or disease. I make no apologies for being a believer in Jesus Christ, therefore as a result of that belief, the material presented in these pages is filled with a multitude of Biblical references which refer to not only healing, but, also passages that speak of God's character, and how He relates to us and works in our lives. For you, the reader, it is important to understand that the truths given in this book are applicable to anyone who is contending against cancer or any other disease or sickness. It makes absolutely no difference if you are a Believer in Christ, Buddhist, Muslim, a non-believer, Atheist, New Age, or of any other religious persuasion, an alcoholic, drug addict, murderer, rapist, or terrorist. The wonderful and absolute truth is that God truly loves you. He does hate our wrong actions, not because they harm or affect Him, but because they cause pain to ourselves and others. The great news is that He truly and unconditionally loves everyone and desires to not only heal everyone, but will do all you allow Him to do to make it happen in your life. God wants to heal you! My prayer is that you will receive your healing as the truths found in this book find a way to enter your heart.

Although this is my story of how cancer was defeated in my life, that is only a small part of this book and is much more than just another story of victory over cancer. During my journey of contending against cancer, I pondered about all of the many so called paradoxes in the failures of some great men and women of faith to be healed. Out of this pondering, the Lord answered many questions which I believe will greatly help you in your journey, not only in contending against sickness or disease, but in many other areas of life. In these pages are also insights and valuable lessons the Lord has revealed in over 40 years of ministry. I believe they will help you greatly in overcoming some major hindrances to healing in your life. This work is also much more than how to be healed from a debilitating sickness, lingering pain, or life threatening disease. Although this book truly did begin as the story on how I defeated cancer, it has somehow morphed into a book which I believe will release truths deep into your heart, which will see you not only healed physically or emotionally, but will propel you into living the life that is promised in God's word. My hope and prayer is that the truths found in these pages will not only build your faith to be healed, but will also give you the faith and courage to pray for others in your day to day life. If you are the one who is contending against cancer or sickness, my prayer is that you will receive your healing even as you are reading this book. With these words, I send you on your journey of healing so you may live a life full of health, free of sickness and pain.

CANCER, THE DREADED WORD

If there is a word that strikes terror and foreboding in the hearts of people, it is the big C word, called cancer. And, to be honest the big pharmaceutical companies and medical establishments do their best to instill that fear in order to keep the dollars rolling in. A good example is convincing women to get yearly mammograms. Unfortunately they neglect to mention (because of the profits involved) that mammograms can cause any existing cancer cells to spread as a result of the radiation and pressure involved. Biopsies can also spread any existing cancer cells. An accurate and much safer pain free alternative to mammograms is Thermography. Unfortunately, whether we like it or not, money drives the health care business more than we know. And that includes alternative health care and the supplement industry. Unfortunately, money often compromises truth in the health industry. The good news in the midst of all the fear concerning cancer and other so called terminal diseases is that they can all be defeated. To be honest, cancer should not strike fear in us any more than a headache or the common cold. For God, the creator of the universe, healing cancer is no more difficult than healing a headache.

All true and permanent healing is a supernatural work of God, which can and should become a natural and normal occurrence in our lives. We were created to live in health all our lives as did Moses.

INSTILLING FEAR KEEPS MONEY FLOWING AND SHAREHOLDERS HAPPY

Doctors are not our enemies. They are a gift from God and are fighting the same enemies of disease and sickness that we contend against. It is true that a small minority of doctors exist who are unprincipled, corrupt, and in the profession strictly for financial benefits, and some are inept and can cause much harm to a patient. However, the overwhelming majority of doctors are good people who became doctors for the purpose of helping people. Multitudes of lives have been saved because of their skill and wisdom. If I broke a leg, was in a car accident or had a ruptured appendix, I would immediately pray for healing, but, if an instant manifestation of healing didn't occur I would go to the hospital. I am not against doctors or hospitals. I firmly believe they are a gift from God, but also believe that God should be our first line of defense, and not plan B if doctors and the medical profession fail to bring results.

My wife and I minister in some poor countries, and since they cannot afford to buy glasses or hearing aids, their only choice is to go blind or deaf. Their hospitals are very inadequate, and as a result, many people who have major problems usually die instead of recover. One hospital we visited was very pitiful. We definitely were not very confident in their ability to help people, especially after we saw they had a funeral home on the property as part of its service.

The people in these situations do not have a plan B. Their only hope is God. When we minister in these countries, we see amazing miracles and high numbers of people healed of serious problems. A recent example of how God is their only hope came from a leader in Fiji who requested a prayer cloth because of some serious physical problems he was having. Like the Apostle Paul in Acts 19:12, I wore a small cloth for a few days, then anointed it with oil and sent it to him. As soon as he placed it on his body, his high blood pressure immediately became normal at 123 over 77, the blurriness in his eyes disappeared, the numbness in his muscles left, and his back pain was instantly healed. No praying, just simple faith to receive the anointing of God from a small piece of cloth.

The reason is that people in poor countries, like my pastor friend, know God is the only plan available which holds any true hope for them, therefore they look to Him in great faith and are instantly healed. In America with our amazing medical technology, cutting edge hospitals and well trained doctors, it's too easy for people to reach for an aspirin, go to the drug store or see a doctor. The result is that our faith has been placed in the medical world instead of in God, making the physical realm our plan A.

Because of our reliance on man's medicine, we look to God only when it seems like the world system is failing us, or like some Believers that I observe, treat God as a part B Medicare supplement or insurance policy.

The idea taught in many churches that God only wants to heal and do miracles among poor nations is absolutely hogwash. It's total ignorance of what the Bible teaches, and even worse, it is an insult to God Himself. God doesn't change His love or His nature from one nation to another. He's the same yesterday and will be the same today and the same tomorrow. You can also be assured that He will be the same God in America as He is in Africa.

Too often people beg God or try to manipulate Him to do something they want and call it prayer. Faith and correct belief are the only true keys to healing! Perhaps what needs to change is our mindset and way of thinking if we desire to see positive results when it comes to healing.

Jesus already paid for our healing when He died on the cross two thousand years ago. Your healing is waiting for you at this very instant as you read these words.

At the time of writing this revision, my wife has been hiding out with the Lord in another location for several weeks, but on her bed are gifts waiting for her to receive. She is unaware they await her, but if she was aware, she wouldn't be begging me to buy those gifts, because she knows they are already hers. To enjoy them, all she has to do is receive them.

Healing is really that simple. But, we need to change some thinking and believing to see it happen in our lives. Further on we will talk about some things that hinder us from receiving what we need.

I want to repeat that I am not against doctors, hospitals or medicine. Luke, who wrote the gospel that bears his name along with the book of Acts was a doctor.

Neither is God against medicine, for without His wisdom, the advances we see in our medical knowledge wouldn't be possible. But, what I, and also believe God would like to see happen, is for us to change the order to where God is our plan A, and for doctors to be our plan B.

Doctors are our friends, however the challenge we face is that they are trapped in a system that really doesn't want to cure cancer or other major illnesses due to the billions of dollars involved. The other major issue with doctors is that the majority of their training has been directed to treating symptoms, and not the root cause of a disease or sickness. This isn't to criticize them, but rather to point out that their ability is limited by their knowledge of what they see in the physical world.

When God heals a person, He heals the root cause and the resulting symptoms. God's way is to bring total healing to the symptoms and the root cause so we can live in health. It isn't God's best for us to spend our life and resources to fight symptoms without dealing with the root causes.

Because the medical profession is mainly trained and equipped to work in the physical realm, they are limited to dealing with the symptoms, and not always able to address the root cause unless God reveals it to them. I am reminded of the woman with the issue of blood in the Bible.

"A woman in the crowd had suffered for

twelve years with constant bleeding. She had suffered a great deal from many doctors, and over the years she had spent everything she had to pay them, but she had gotten no better. In fact, she had gotten worse. Then she heard about Jesus." (Mark 5:25-27) NLT

Did you know that Jesus will heal you and never send you a bill or ask you whether you have insurance or Medicare supplement insurance, before He agrees to treat you as most doctors and hospitals do? God works both in the spiritual realm which deals with the true source, and in the physical realm in order to produce lasting healing, whether by an instant miracle or gradual healing over hours, a few days or several weeks.

There is always a spiritual component that's the root cause of all sickness and disease. This is why dealing with just the physical realm often leads to failure. Before I begin my cancer story, it would be good to give some background that may help you to relate and better understand, and how to apply what you are about to read to your own situation and life.

Sometimes it's helpful and easier for others to accept answers and thoughts from those who have gone through similar struggles and circumstances, rather than from those who have never had to deal with a major trauma such as disease or sickness.

Cancer was no stranger to my life. My own mother died from a long battle with cancer that began in her big toe. They cut her toe off, along with ministering chemo and radiation therapy. But, they couldn't stop the cancer from spreading. They continued to amputate multiple times, using more chemo and radiation, until there was no more to cut away after the cancer reached her hip. She finally succumbed after many years of much pain and suffering, both physically and emotionally.

Besides my mother, cancer has taken two aunts, an uncle, a brother and a wife, so I can say as mentioned previously that cancer is no stranger to my life. The sad aspect is that although my mother's battle with cancer occurred nearly seventy years ago, the medical establishment is still using the same protocols. Their answer is still surgery, radiation and chemo therapy, despite the fact there are some successful alternative therapies that don't cause the debilitating and deadly side effects.

Even worse is that they have no better results today than they had with my mother. Of course this is contrary to what the medical establishment and drug companies want us to believe through the manipulation of statistics making things appear better than they really are.

Many oncologists would greatly hesitate to give their own wives and children radiation or chemo therapy because they know the horrible side effects, not to mention the end results. I recently heard of a well-known minister who was contending against cancer, and went through the normal route of chemo and radiation treatment. The prognosis was that he only had a few months to live even with their treatment.

In the midst of this the Lord sent a woman to him to pray for him and he was instantly healed. He went back to the doctor to confirm his healing, which was indeed confirmed that he no longer had cancer, however the doctor informed him that because of the radical doses of chemo and radiation, that even though his cancer was gone, he guaranteed this minister would die within six months due to the radical treatments.

Let me test your intelligence. Is it wisdom to submit to that kind of treatment if you were guaranteed to die from the treatment even if they stopped the cancer? The happy ending for this minister is that when he was healed by Jesus, he was healed from both the cancer and the side effects of the radical chemo and radiation treatments.

God always has the last word! As a matter of fact He appears to love impossible odds. Just read some of the impossible odds Israel faced when leaving Egypt, when they were in the desert, and also when they went into the promised land where they had to fight many battles when they were tremendously outnumbered. It seems God loves to show up and show off, and more important, He would love to show up and show off in your situation.

The other aspect is that doctors and the medical profession absolutely know they can't cure cancer or other major diseases. All they can do is attempt to slow a disease process down so the body has a fighting chance to heal itself. What they often call remission is just another way to say they have managed to slow the cancer growth sufficiently in the hopes that the body is in a better position to heal itself. Sometimes they are successful, but often they aren't.

As mentioned, the main challenge the medical profession faces is that they are only able to treat the symptoms and not the root cause. You can pick an apple tree bare, but the next year, the tree will once again produce more apples. The only way to prevent a tree from continually bearing fruit is to kill the roots so nutrients cannot enter the tree. No roots = no tree = no fruit.

Although, cancer wreaked havoc in my family lineage and in my personal life, I have never had a fear of cancer because of my belief in a good God. I have too often witnessed the miracles He has worked in the lives of countless people with cancer and other major diseases. Seeing what He has done in others keeps me believing that He is good and desires to heal us.

In the process of ministering healing prayer to people, I have witnessed many amazing miracles such as instant healing of cancer, broken backs, club feet instantly straightened, endometriosis healed, and my own broken leg, besides the cancer the enemy tried to destroy me with.

God desires to heal us because He loves us and wants to care for us in all areas of our lives. A few years ago while ministering in Israel, I prayed for an Eritrean woman who desperately wanted to have children, but had gone through a hysterectomy which ended her hopes for children. But God always has the last word! When I returned the next year, she showed me her beautiful new baby boy.

Key #1: She was instantly healed, but it still took nine months for it to manifest. She didn't feel anything when I prayed and could have walked away believing nothing had happened. But, she kept her faith that she was healed even though the manifestation didn't come until some weeks had passed and she began to see the signs of her healing.

Key #2: If she had walked away believing nothing had happened, she would have lost her miracle. Sometimes our healing may take time to see in the natural, so we must stay in faith believing we were healed. I will cover this more thoroughly further on.

While so many healings and miracles were spectacular and temp me to talk about some of them, it's needful and more important to concentrate on the subject of cancer. A cancer miracle that greatly impacted me and gave me great faith to believe it's God will to heal everyone occurred many years ago in Costa Rico.

I was speaking on the goodness of God and at the close of the service a young woman came up for prayer. She had a cancer growth in the roof of her mouth so large it prevented her from speaking or even closing her mouth. Besides the constant pain she had to endure, they had to puree all her food into a liquid and spoon it into her mouth because she couldn't close her mouth sufficiently to chew. I never had a chance to even pray for her, because as soon as I touched her the growth disappeared before our eyes and all the pain immediately left.

When you witness such a miracle it removes all doubt that Jesus desires to heal people today just as much as He did when He walked the earth two thousand years ago.

Seeing God work in miraculous ways through the years not only strengthens my faith, but at the same time grieves me because of some who teach that He no longer heals today, or that it may not be His will to heal you, or some other variation of how He may not want you to be healed. The truth is that we serve a loving God Who is only capable of love and continually works on our behalf.

"You are good, and what you do is good; teach

me your decrees." *(Psalm 119:68)* NKJV.

Decrees are the truths God wants us to believe about Him. He wants us to believe His Word, that He is good and that He only does good. There is a major flaw with the belief of some churches, which teach that God no longer heals today. Their thinking is grounded on a belief that the dispensation of miracles and healing ended after the 12 apostles died. It's based on the belief that healing and miracles only occurred to establish the early church, therefore are no longer needed because the church is now established.

It doesn't take an Einstein to see that the church may have been established or started, but is presently far from being what God desires. The fact is that history reveals the church has gone backwards in many areas. We desperately need the power of the early church, including healing and miracles, if we the church are to truly become what Jesus desires for His body.

A greater truth is that **there never was a time or dispensation of healing and**

miracles! There is only a God of healing and miracles, Who works miracles in all ages. He is a God who never has and never will change. Healing and miracles are signs and a demonstration of God's character of love and compassion. If God changes and no longer does miracles He would no longer be God. He would be an unpredictable and undependable being who we could never trust because we would never know what He would do next.

If God healed in one age or dispensation, He will heal now, because He is still the same God of love and compassion! Jesus was the earthly revelation of His Father, Who is the source of all healing.

"I have glorified You on the earth. I have finished the work *which You have given me to do." (John 17:4)* NKJV.

Everyone knows and believes that Jesus died on the cross to redeem us from sin, which was a major work, but this particular verse is not speaking of His work on the cross, because His crucifixion had not yet taken place. This passage is speaking of a work that Jesus fulfilled before He went to the cross. The work He is referring to is how He perfectly revealed and represented the love and compassion of His Heavenly Father as He healed and ministered to people.

"The Son can do nothing of Himself, but what He sees the Father do; for whatever He does, the Son also does in like manner." (John 5:19-20) NKJV.

Everything Jesus did during His earthly ministry, including His death on the cross was to do His Father's will, so mankind could know and understand the amazing unconditional love and compassion God has for His creation. Besides the above mentioned spectacular cancer miracle, I have witnessed the most amazing miracles and healings in countless people, which to this day still keeps me in awe of our loving Father and God.

In keeping with my healing story, an important aspect is for you to understand that even though I believed in miracles, it didn't prevent the devil from attacking me with cancer.

Just because we believe God heals and that miracles are for today doesn't always prevent the enemy from attacking us with cancer or any other disease. We are in a war with a relentless enemy so we shouldn't be surprised with his attacks.

It's no surprise that the devil hates God with a twisted and evil passion, but he can't get to God, so he attacks the ones God loves and the ones who love God. Like it or not you are the bullseye in satan's rifle scope! We are at war with our enemy and God's enemy. The good news is that we fight with spiritual weapons that have been designed by God to win every battle.

I refuse to confess, as some say, that we may lose a few battles, but will win the war. **With God, we can and will win every battle and the war.** As the Word of Gods says, we must equip ourselves with God's weapons, stand our ground and fight. The only other option is to desert God's army, but you won't like the results, because deserters will be shot by the enemy.

It would be good to listen to what the apostle Peter said.

"The devil walks about like a roaring lion, seeking who he may devour." (1 Peter 5:8) NKJV

In the wild, a lion knows that if he can get a sheep or other animal to desert the herd, he will sit down to a thanksgiving feast. If we become passive by denying the devil exists or that he won't attack us, deny demons exist, ignore them, believe they cannot oppress or attack believers, or give up the fight, we are guaranteed to be devoured. We have only one option and that's to fight, and surrender no ground until we win. I will speak more on this, but just know that we carry the power and authority of God to trample on the enemy.

We can expect the enemy to always look for opportunities to attack us, but we need not fear. God and the devil have one thing in common. Neither God or satan will ever change. God is always good and satan is always evil.

"The thief comes only to steal, kill, and

destroy; but, I have come that you may have life, and have it to the full." (John 10:10) NIV.

The good news is that we can expect to have victory over the enemy's attacks and to have life to the full, because Jesus came to destroy the works of the enemy and give us life.

"The devil has been sinning from the beginning. The reason the Son of God appeared was to destroy the works of the devil." (1 John 3:8) ESV

The young woman I prayed for in Israel was instantly healed, but it took nine months to fully manifest. Just because manifestation of healing doesn't instantly appear doesn't mean it didn't happen. Jesus already destroyed the works of satan on the cross in the invisible realm, but we often have to fight or contend to see it come into the natural realm. But that doesn't change the truth that we have already been healed 2000 years ago when Jesus shed His blood on the cross.

"He took away the weapons of the powers and

authorities. He made a public show of them. He won the battle over them by dying on the cross." (Colossians 2:15) NIRV

MY STORY

My story began at Bethel Church in Redding California. Bethel Church is well known as a healing center, where countless people have come from all over the world for prayer, and have been healed of cancer and other terminal diseases. After resigning as pastor of a church in central Pennsylvania, we moved to Redding, California. I enrolled in Bethel's school of supernatural ministry, became involved in two inner healing ministries, facilitated a home group, and ministered in Bethel's healing room where the most amazing miracles happened weekly. To say I was busy and deeply involved in ministry would be a major understatement.

In the midst of this busy time, in January of 2009, we discovered my wife had stage four stomach and esophagus cancer. Our first action was for her to receive healing prayer and to believe for a miracle, because we had always made God our plan A, and not plan

B.

We also did what we could in the natural realm. When this discovery came, I immediately discontinued all involvement in ministry in order to concentrate on doing everything we could to defeat the cancer that was attacking her body.

In the natural realm, after much research, we also decided to enter alternative treatment, as conventional treatment offered a success rate of less than two percent for this type of cancer. The treatment was successful in that the cancer was almost completely eradicated to less than five percent remaining. However, at the time she was also dealing with a weak heart. And, due to pressure from large amounts of fluid that had built up around an already overworked heart, she went home to her Jesus in June of 2009.

There are far too many details of how God was working and was in the midst of this ordeal to relate at this time. It's sufficient to say we both were amazed with our wonderful Lord's care and goodness in our midst as we journeyed through the trial.

In the midst of her battle with cancer the enemy never succeeded in diminishing my belief and faith that God is a loving and good God and that He desires to heal everyone. If anything, it served to increase my determination to trust God in the midst of trials no matter how things looked like in the natural realm.

There is always the temptation to become bitter and blame God for not healing a person, or blame ourselves for not having "more faith" or "not doing enough" or "not doing the right things." Our enemy will always look for opportunities to tempt us to hate or blame God and walk away from Him. We will address some of his tactics further on.

The reality is that we'll always be under attack from the enemy, but what matters is what we believe and how we react in the midst of our trials and his temptations. It's always our choice to either give up on God or press in to Him in trust and faith.

After my wife's death, I once again

became deeply immersed in ministry. As mentioned earlier, I was involved with a healing heart ministry of Bethel church, and during a mini conference we were conducting, I met a brilliant medical doctor from Canada, with whom I became friends.

He was very successful with his own clinic in Canada, where he mainly dealt with cancer. However, he soon became disillusioned with the normal protocols of surgery, radiation and chemo therapy. Because of the lack of genuine results and all the serious negative effects of normal medical treatments, he became involved with alternative cancer treatments.

Unfortunately his move into alternative treatments soon caused some unexpected experiences. In the midst of operating his clinic, he developed many supplements and protocols that were highly effective in defeating cancer. However, because of his success in treating cancer, he also soon came under attack by the pharmaceutical and medical establishments. He wasn't only harassed, but had his clinic destroyed twice and literally feared for his life. These unexpected attacks caused him to move to the United States. This isn't unusual for it has also happened many times in our own country.

PHARMACEUTICAL COMPANIES ARE IN BUSINESS TO MAKE MONEY, NOT CURE DISEASES

Forget all the commercials that advertise so many miracle or the many wonder drugs offered for numerous sicknesses and diseases, along with the sad looks on people that are replaced with smiles after using their products. The pharmaceutical companies, whether large or small, as well as some medical establishments make billions of dollars at the expense of hurting people. The sad fact is that they are in business to make money, not to cure diseases. There is nothing wrong with companies making a reasonable profit, but there is a major problem when greed takes over and a reasonable profit becomes an exorbitant profit at the expense of hurting people.

Although supplements are a safer and much cheaper alternative to prescription drugs, caution needs to be exercised in several areas. It's up to you to do your research to make sure the product fits your need and most important they contain quality ingredients. Lastly, the last few years has brought a plethora of snake oil merchants, where their products are of dubious value. Except in the case of God, if it's too good to be true, it's probably a scam of some sorts. My wife and I are strong proponents of needed supplements because of the huge lack of nutrients in our modern diets, but we use wisdom and choose wisely. Next is the importance of whether you actually need them or will a change in lifestyle and eating habits solve your problem or accomplish the same goal?

Greedy supplement companies are springing up every day on the internet promising things they cannot possibly deliver, and like the big drug companies are money making machines at the expense of your health and your hard earned money.

My medical friend who came to the United States was an absolutely brilliant man, and had the ability to look at a person's facial skin tones and detect problems and diseases that were subsequently verified through further testing.

One day in the spring of 2010, we were at lunch and I could see he was studying my face, which was a little unnerving, since I could tell by his expression that he was concerned about something he was seeing. He then asked me to begin taking some supplements which he had developed.

A week or so later, he gave me some additional supplements along with some food protocols that he wanted me to follow. After another week he said that he wanted me to get blood work done to test for cancer. His observations were correct as the tests showed that I indeed had cancer. In the following weeks, he put me on a strict diet, along with various therapies to fight the cancer onslaught upon my body, which was beginning to really affect me physically.

By the end of summer in 2010 the monthly tests kept getting worse and I went from weighing 165 pounds to around

125 pounds. Normally, I was used to a maximum of about 6-7 hours of sleep but during this time I would sleep 10-12 hours, yet on arising it seemed like I needed to go back to bed. It felt like a plug was pulled draining away all my energy, and it took sheer will power just to make it through each day.

You need to understand that in the midst of this trial, I never stopped believing that God was a loving God Who desired everyone to be healed including me. However, as I learned firsthand, just because we believe God is good and believe in healing, it doesn't prevent the devil from attacking us.

I was reminded of a book I had read many years ago, that portrayed exactly what I was going through. The author was a great man of faith, yet he was dying from some disease. The title of the book was, "I believed in healing, yet I was dying." It is very likely that many people can relate to what he and I were experiencing. Hopefully, as you read, you will find some answers to what appears to be paradoxes in our lives.

Like the experiences of other healing ministers, in the midst of my own battle, I was seeing tremendous miracles as I prayed for others. Talk about a paradox! I was seeing God move in great ways in the lives of others, yet victory over my own battle against cancer seemed allusive. It was like someone who drowns in the process of saving another person from drowning. Battles can be real and heart wrenching, can't they?

Although I'm not a Catholic I flew from California to a monastery in New Mexico in late summer. I not only went to get a break from all that I was going through, but also to see a woman I was pursuing, who became my wife two years later. Pursuing her seemed to be another paradox since my body appeared to be losing the battle.

However, looking back and seeing her as my future wife also gave me hope and a major reason to continue to fight for life and not give up.

WE ALL NEED A REASON AND PURPOSE TO LIVE

We all need a reason and purpose to live. I have often observed that when some people retire they end up dying soon after because they no longer had a reason to live. Without a purpose or reason to wake up in the morning, many people often don't wake up. Although everything in the natural seemed to indicate my death was near I had absolutely no fear. How can we fear if we know we're going home to a loving Father? At the same time I loved life, and didn't want to go before my time.

Deep inside my heart, I knew God still had a destiny for me on this earth that needed to be finished. The trip to the monastery also proved important as God used it to reinforce a valuable spiritual lesson. It's a proven medical fact that oxygen is an enemy of cancer cells, and that the closer to sea level you can be, the better to fight cancer because of the higher oxygen content in the atmosphere. My home at the time was in Redding California which is somewhere between 400 and 500 feet above sea level at its highest point. In the natural realm it was a good place to live to contend against cancer because of the higher levels of oxygen, compared to the lower levels at higher elevations. The monastery in New Mexico is around sixty-five hundred feet above sea level which in the natural is not a good place to fight cancer because of the lower oxygen levels. Now, here is part of the spiritual lesson that was reinforced. After a week at the monastery my energy began to increase which was contrary to what should have occurred. Perhaps part of it can be explained due to the fact I was able to spend time with my future wife who was and is the love of my life.

The other aspect was due to the spiritual setting where I could spend time with the Lord without all the interruptions and busyness of my normal life.

This particular monastery is located thirteen miles off the main road at the end of a dead end canyon with no cell service or electricity other than solar panels. It's also a silent order, meaning there's no talking allowed except in a designated small library building. The peacefulness and silence is a breath of fresh air. Too often we're so busy in the midst of a noisy and frantic world, that it's a major hindrance to hearing and communing with our Heavenly Father.

CANCER AND ALL DISEASES ARE FIRST AND FORMOST A SPIRITUAL BATTLE

The spiritual lesson I learned, proved without a doubt that cancer as well as all diseases are first and foremost a major spiritual battle. This isn't to minimize the physical aspect, but all too often we concentrate on the physical first instead of the spiritual and lose far too many battles as a result.

At the end of my stay at the monastery, although I didn't feel well by any stretch of the imagination, there was an obvious difference for the better. It was what took place when I arrived back in Redding, California that I was taken completely by surprise. What occurred proved beyond a shadow of a doubt the spiritual battles we face when contending against any type of disease, sickness, emotional problem, or other issues for that matter.

Bethel Church, as previously mentioned is known all over the world as a healing center, where tremendous healings and miracles take place on a daily basis. But, along with that, there's an equally important truth that we should always keep in mind. Anywhere God is moving, you can be sure the enemy of our spirits, souls and bodies will also be there to contend against what God is doing.

In many circles, people talk about portals, thin places or open heavens where it is easier to connect with God. While this is true, the greater truth is that any location where there are open portals, thin places or open heavens, you will also find strong activity of the enemy from]the second heaven

Two places besides Bethel come to mind where we have personally experienced where both God's angels and satan's demons are active. Moravian Falls in North Carolina and Jerusalem. It's no secret that God and the devil have clashed over Jerusalem for thousands of years and it won't end until Jesus comes back. Moravian

Falls is the location of Prayer Mountain where it's claimed that the Moravians prayed for twenty-four hours a day, seven days a week, 365 days a year for a hundred years. If you are even slightly spiritually attuned, you can feel the presence of God and angels, along with feeling the presence of the enemy. There are many other places, but these two are major playing fields for both God and satan that we have personally experienced.

There was so much spiritual activity of both realms in Moravian falls that Bob Jones, a prophetic voice to the church, had trouble sleeping, and had to move because there was too much spiritual activity in the invisible realm. And many others also reported having the same problem.

The Redding airport is very small and they only have thirty seat planes which meant you entered and exited the planes from the tarmac. As mentioned, I was feeling fairly well, but the **exact instant my foot physically touched the ground** upon exiting the plane, it was like someone suddenly pulled a plug out of me. I was totally shocked as I felt all my energy instantly drained from my body and was back to the same weak condition as when I had left Redding. In the natural, coming back to near sea level, I should have felt better instead of worse. Because the opposite happened, it revealed the tremendous spiritual warfare in our lives. This truth applies not just in contending against physical diseases but also applies to our everyday spiritual and emotional life.

We must never forget that we are in a war that will never end until we go home to Father God or when Jesus comes back. The enemy doesn't go away simply because he is defeated in one battle. He understands better than we do, that it's a war we must win, not just win one battle.

WE MUST NEVER FORGET WE ARE IN THE MIDST OF SPIRITUAL BATTLES

Jesus discovered this when His temptations in the garden were concluded.

*"When the devil had ended every temptation, he departed from Him, until **a more opportune time.**"* (my emphasis). *(Luke 4:10)* NKJV.

If satan looked for more opportune times to attack Jesus, you can be sure he will do the same with us. Although we're in the midst of warfare it's vital to keep in mind that we don't have to fear because we have Jesus, the overcomer living in us and among us.

Faith should be our banner, and never fear. There is a great acrostic that speaks about the difference between fear and faith. Fear is *"false effects appearing real,"* But faith is *"free access into the heavenlies."*

Before I relate my miracle, I would like to

speak of some truths or principles that are very important for you to know if you're in a spiritual or physical battle. When I spoke of my doctor friend who began to notice some things in me physically, I allowed my friendship and respect for him as a medical professional to affect my heart and mind.

This is a very important point because the medical profession has trained doctors to act as gods before us so we don't question their assessments or not follow their advice. This can be beneficial for helping us to follow directions that are meant to help us, but it can also be very detrimental at times, because it can produce unwanted outcomes in our pursuit of healing whether physically or emotionally.

WE CAN UNKNOWINGLY ALLOW WORDS OF OTHERS TO NEGATIVELY IMPACT OUR LIFE

Too often we allow a prognosis or destructive words of doctors, friends, family, or others that we respect or those we are close with, to negatively impact us in our soul and spirit. My friend never tried to act as a god to me, but I respected not only his ability, but more importantly, honored him as a friend who truly cared for me. Therefore, I allowed his words to have a greater impact on me in ways that were not seen at the time.

I want to emphasize that he didn't knowingly or unknowingly desire to negatively impact me with his words. The fault was on my part in receiving his words as truth, instead of just hearing him relate physical facts. We must always remember that no matter how factual something sounds or appears, we must allow God's truth to always drive our hearts and minds, and override any facts we may hear.

"What you say (and the words of others that we receive) (my insert) *can preserve or destroy life, because you will receive the consequences of your words" (Proverbs 18:21)* GNB

*"You are taken as in a net by the words of your mouth, the sayings of **your lips** have overcome you"* (my Emphasis) *(Proverbs 6:2)* BBE

Looking back, I believe our friendship was perhaps more deadly than if I had gone and listened to a normal medical doctor. Even worse, was the fact that I knew better, and constantly cautioned others about never receiving negative words from anyone no matter who they are.

Even with all my experience and training, it shows how sly the enemy is and how easily it is to allow our hearts to receive facts as truth. After having ministered to countless people dealing with physical issues I have seen how impactful doctors, friends and family, who mean only the best, can often have a very negative and sometimes deadly effect through the words they speak to us or over us.

Even though they have good intentions, their words can have a much greater effect, when it comes from someone we love or respect. I'm not saying what my friend saw in me was wrong, or that his diagnosis was wrong. What I'm saying is that his words spoke deep into my soul and heart and empowered the enemy because I received his words in my heart as truth rather than just facts.

A word becomes a curse upon us physically and spiritually anytime it doesn't agree with God's Word, His Nature or His Character.

"As a man thinks in his heart, so is he." (Proverbs 23:7) NKJV.

To rephrase this passage to address this area, we could say, "whatever thoughts or words are placed into our hearts and minds, whether by others or ourselves will cause us to eventually become what has been placed there."

"Guard your heart above all else for it determines the course of your life." (Proverbs 4:23) NLT

Solomon's words in this passage are just another way to say we will become or produce in the spiritual and/or physical realm what is residing in our hearts. Because of our friendship, I had allowed my friend to place in my heart an outcome which I didn't want, nor did God want. God's desire is for us to have full life, not sickness or premature death. Proverbs 23:7 in The Good News Bible is even stronger in its warning over our thoughts.

"Be careful how you think; because your life is shaped by your thoughts." (Proverbs 23:7) GNB

That is why it is so extremely important for us to not receive words and thoughts from others which may be detrimental to us spiritually or physically, no matter whom it comes from or how good their intentions may be. We can be kind and listen to their words as facts, but we do not have to receive their words as truth.

To be honest most of the people in our lives desire to help us, not do us harm. But, that doesn't mean we should receive everything they offer us. Someone once said, "just because someone rings your door bell or calls your phone, doesn't mean you have to open the door or answer your phone." I get numerous spam calls on my cell phone, but if I don't recognize it or if it isn't in my contact list, I ignore it, and if they don't leave a voice mail, I block and delete it. We should treat a lot of words we get from people like spam calls. If it isn't in God's contact list of His truth and His nature, we should Block and Delete!

We need to be proactive in screening, and rejecting anything that does not line up with God's Word, His Nature or His Character. To be brutally honest, with all the emphasis on eating properly, we tend to be more careful about what we put into our stomachs than what we put in our hearts. But this should not be the normal procedure for a follower of Jesus Christ.

"Take heed what you hear for with the same measure you use (or receive), *it will*

be measured (or given) to you and to you who hear (or receive), *more will be given to you."* (my inserts) *(Mark 4:24)* NKJV.

The principle in this verse is that if we receive negative words as truth the enemy will make sure we will hear and receive more of the same words to our detriment. I don't apologize for speaking so strongly on this, as it's a major way the enemy brings destruction into our lives.

"Death and life are in the power of the tongue and those who love it will eat its fruit." (Proverbs 18:21) NKJV.

Beware: Our own negative words that we speak carry more weight and have a far greater effect than the words of others. Everyone believes that the way of others is the wrong way to do things, and that our way is the correct way. The truth is that we trust our own words and opinions much more than the words and opinions of others.

Whenever we receive negative words from others or ourselves, there is also a tendency to rehearse them in our minds or even speak them out loud, and thereby increase their negative effect. Words received into our heart, whether the words of others and especially our own words will bring forth either fruit of death or fruit of life. We need to be careful, not only of what others speak into our lives, but we also need to be very careful of the words that we speak into the lives of others as well as the words we speak into our own lives.

Someone said that words will become thoughts, the thoughts will become our beliefs, and our beliefs will produce either good or bad results. Remember the apple tree? It's the root, or in this instance, what we receive as truth that will become a belief in our hearts, which will then determine the kind of fruit we bear, whether in the spiritual or physical realm.

WE ALONE CAN DECIDE
TO RECEIVE WORDS OF
LIFE OR DEATH

We alone have the responsibility and the ability to receive or reject words that will negatively affect us. My present wife has a wonderful saying that came from John G. Lake, a great healing evangelist in the early 1900's. *"what we behold, we will attract to us, and therefore we will soon become that which we behold."* This holds true in all areas of our lives, therefore we need to diligently guard and refuse to receive any words that have the potential to produce anything in our lives that we don't want, no matter if they come from others or ourselves.

SATAN ALWAYS COMES TO DISPUTE AND STEAL WHAT GOD SPEAKS TO US

Satan always comes to dispute what God speaks to us. He did it in the garden with Adam and Eve, with Jesus in the desert, and he'll do it with us. At the baptism of Jesus, the heaven was opened and the Holy Spirit descended in bodily form like a dove upon Him and God's spoke from heaven to voice His love and approval for Jesus.

"You are my beloved Son and in You I am well pleased." (Luke 3:21-22) NKJV.

The very next thing that happened was that Jesus was driven into the wilderness, where the devil challenged God's Word to Him.

"If you are the Son of God turn this stone into bread."

We need to be mindful that if Jesus was

tested on what His Father said to Him, we can be sure the enemy will always test a word or truth that we receive from God. This is exactly what happened to me. Satan tried to steal words that God had spoken to me, just like he did with Jesus and Adam and Eve.

When I returned from the monastery, I went further downhill, and by the end of September if something didn't drastically and quickly change, my life on earth would soon end. However, as someone once said, God always has the last word. It's quite amazing to me that God seems to enjoy coming on the scene at the last moment to laugh in satan's face.

"God in heaven merely laughs! He is amused by all their puny plans." (Psalms 2:4) TLB.

In October I awoke with the Lord reminding me of a vision He had given me in the night back in January of the same year. In the vision the Lord said that He was giving me back twenty years. Although there were many other aspects to the vision, the important part was that I knew He was speaking about my physical or health realm.

SATAN WILL ALWAYS TEST GOD'S WORD TO US

Just like with Jesus after receiving His Father's word, the devil immediately tested and tried to abort what the Lord had told me in the vision. I have to confess that I had forgotten what the Lord had spoken to me. You're probably thinking, how could I forget something so vital to my life? The truth is that the attack didn't come until after several months of receiving the vision. Then in the busyness of ministry and life, I totally forgot the vision and allowed the enemy to win some battles. What can I say? I am human.

The good news for you is that if I can forget something as important as His vision to me and still be healed, there is great hope for you. God works on behalf of imperfect people, not those who have it all together. The great news is that God's Word to us always stays true, never loses power, and will always perform what it was sent to do.

*"As the rain and the snow come down from heaven, and do not return to it without watering the earth and making it bud and flourish, so that it yields seed for the sower and bread for the eater, so is my word that goes out from my mouth: **It will not return to me empty, but will accomplish what I desire and achieve the purpose for which I sent it.**"* (my emphasis) *(Isaiah 55:10-11)* NIV.

Here is a very important aspect to my healing. A lot of times when things happen in our lives we often undertake major warfare against the enemy, which isn't wrong in any way, and many times a very important ingredient for us to achieve victory.

Please understand that I'm not against warfare as I firmly believe in it, and live with a wife who is an amazing intercessor. But, what I do want to emphasize is that we often pray from our heads and emotions instead of from our hearts.

I heard a minister once say that God doesn't listen to what we pray. Of course when I heard that, my first thought was that he was wrong, because the Bible says over and over again that God not only hears us, but even knows what's going on in our hearts and minds.

"The word of God is alive and active. Sharper than any double-edged sword, it penetrates even to dividing soul and spirit, joints and marrow; it judges the thoughts and attitudes of the heart. Nothing in all creation is hidden from God's sight. Everything is uncovered and laid bare before the eyes of Him to whom we must give account." (Hebrews 4:12-13) NIV.

But, what the minister was trying to say is that God hears what our heart is saying, as opposed to just the words of our mouth if they aren't in agreement. Faith that moves mountains must come from our hearts, not just from our heads or our mouths.

"With the heart one believes unto righteousness (believes what is true and right), *and with the mouth confession is made unto* (our healing) *salvation."* (my inserts) *(Romans 10:10)* NKJV.

The Greek word for salvation is an all-inclusive term that means much more than salvation of our spirits. It carries a meaning of salvation, protection, deliverance, provision and healing. God's idea of salvation is for the total person, body, soul and spirit. God's idea is to fix everything that is broken, and to provide anything that is missing for us to have His concept or His kind of life.

However, genuine salvation or healing only comes when our spoken words line up with what's in our hearts. Without lining up with what is in our heart, we're just speaking empty and faithless words from our heads, not true words of faith from our heart. That's a major reason why some people's lives never change after speaking the so called "sinner's prayer."

It all begins in and must come from the heart. That is also why there are times when our prayers don't seem to accomplish anything. It's because our hearts and words are not in agreement. My cancer experience is a good example of how what I believed in my head was different from what I believed in my heart.

When the Lord reminded me of the vision, I didn't pray, rebuke the cancer, nor did I rebuke or yell at the devil. I really didn't even think or dwell on it until many weeks later. But true faith rose up in my heart as I came into agreement with what the Lord spoke to me in the vision which He had given me in January. Because faith came into my heart, within three days I was cancer free, back to normal strength and energy, and regained the lost weight within three weeks. That was nearly 12 years ago at the time of this book revision, and I'm going strong and living in the truth of that vision. But, far more important, is that out of the lessons learned, I am living in the truth of His Word.

There are two very important truths about my healing. First, you need to understand that **the vision didn't heal me.** What healed me was **faith in God and faith in His Word** which came through the vision. The second great truth is that it doesn't matter how His Word comes to us, whether from a passage in the Bible, a prophetic word, a word of knowledge, or from a dream or vision. What is important is that the word we receive originates from Him.

When a UPS driver delivers a package, the value is found in what the package contains, not in the delivery method or the driver. In the end, we shouldn't care how faith and healing comes as long as it comes. What we allow to be put into our hearts is far more important than what's in our minds. Our minds may not always think or believe according to truth, but it's our hearts that will determine how we live our lives.

Although Romans 10:8-10 is used primarily for leading people to salvation, it was never meant to be restricted only to the redemption of our spirits, but was meant to apply to our whole being of body, soul and spirit. The death of Jesus on the cross was God's method to redeem and fix everything that is broken or missing in our life, spiritually, physically and emotionally.

"The word is near you; it is in your mouth and in your heart, that is, the message concerning faith that we proclaim. If you declare with

*your mouth, Jesus is Lord, and **believe in your heart** that God raised him from the dead, you will be saved. For it is with your heart that you believe and are justified, and it is with your mouth that you profess your faith* (profess what is in your heart) *and are* (healed) *saved."* (my emphasis and insert). *(Romans 10:8-10)* NKJV.

"Do not conform to the pattern of this world, but be transformed by the renewing of your mind. Then you will be able to test and approve what God's will is, his good, pleasing and perfect will." (Romans 12:2) NIV.

The intent of this passage in Romans is not to fill our minds with knowledge. It didn't work for the Pharisees and it won't work for us. What God wants is to bring His truth into our hearts and to bring our minds into agreement with our spirits and our hearts because God doesn't want our minds divided from our hearts.

THE FAITH IN OUR HEARTS
MUST EQUAL THE FAITH
IN OUR WORDS

In the midst of my trial, much time was spent pondering some of the seemingly paradoxes or tensions we see in the area of healing. To be honest, there are some questions that will never be answered this side of heaven, but the one truth we must never let go of is that God is always good.

"You are good and do only good; teach me Your ways." (or teach me to believe you are good and only do good) (my insert) *(Psalms 119:68)* NLT.

There is no question in my mind that the devil continually attacks two areas when it comes to healing. First, He's constantly attacking the veracity of God's word just as he did in the garden with Eve. If satan can get us to question God or His promises, he can destroy our faith to receive what we need in our lives. Satan works hard to have us believe that God cannot be trusted to do what He says He already did or will do for us.

The second area is that he goes to great lengths to convince people it isn't always God's will to heal them. One of his lies is that if God wanted to heal them they would already be healed. Another of his lies is that there must be something wrong with them which is stopping God from healing them or wanting to heal them. The implication is that we have no value or are not worthy enough for God to even want to heal us.

Although there are some hindrances that can prevent us from receiving God's healing which we will address shortly. They have nothing to do with our worthiness or with God wanting to heal us. God wants to heal us so much that He sent His Son to die on the cross for our healing.

Another very successful tactic of satan is to point out how great men or women of God who believed in healing, yet they themselves died from cancer or another major disease. The devil knows that if he can succeed in destroying leaders or people who appear to have great faith with cancer, heart attacks or other major diseases, he can have a much greater effect on the faith of those who follow those leaders.

You can be sure that he'll try to convince you that healing isn't for everyone by using a leader's death from cancer or other disease as an example. He uses them as an example to place words or thoughts in our hearts and minds to destroy our faith and our view of God such as, "what makes you think you can be healed, if this great person of faith, who had thousands praying for them, couldn't get healed?" Or, "what makes you think it's God's will to heal you if it wasn't His will to heal this great person of faith?"

The list of the thoughts and words he uses to destroy our faith can vary and be endless as some of you well know from your own experience. Not only does satan attempt to plant those kinds of thoughts in us, but all too often, he uses incorrect and wrong messages from pulpits and ministries to support the idea that it isn't God's will to heal everyone.   Satan isn't only the author of sickness and disease, but his number one goal besides preventing you from receiving your healing is to get you to doubt God's word, and to destroy your belief that God loves and cares about you.

We can "say" God is good and "say" we believe that He wants to heal us, but when voices from the enemy of our souls come with lies from many sources, our faith for healing and good thoughts about God can evaporate. The result is we begin to question God's love and desire to care for us.

The Bible speaks very clearly that satan is our enemy, not God. That Jesus came to die on the cross for our sins is an absolute truth. But, His death on the cross is in the context of a much bigger picture and assignment. His mission on earth was to represent a loving God whom the world lost sight of. As Jesus healed and set people free, the Bible makes it very clear that God is good and was behind all that Jesus did.

"Lord, show us the Father, and it is sufficient

for us. Jesus said to him, have I been with you so long, and yet you have not known Me, Philip? He who has seen Me has seen the Father; so how can you say, Show us the Father? Do you not believe that I am in the Father, and the Father in Me? The words that I speak to you I do not speak on My own authority; but the Father who dwells in Me does the works. Believe Me that I am in the Father and the Father in Me, or else believe Me for the sake of the works themselves." (John 14:8-11) NKJV.

Jesus clearly said in many passages that He only did what He saw the Father doing, and that He came to earth to reveal His heavenly Father to the world. He also made it clear that He came to undo what satan was doing.

"The devil has been sinning since the beginning, but the Son of God came to destroy the works of the devil." (1 John 3:8) NLT.

Please note that although the devil will one day be thrown into the lake of fire, it wasn't the present task of Jesus when He was on earth. Jesus came for the sole purpose of revealing the Father through His ministering to people and to destroy the works or effects the devil has on mankind through the cross.

"The thief comes only in order to steal, kill, and destroy. I have come in order that you might have life in all its fullness." (John 10:10) GNB.

As mentioned earlier, salvation includes far more than redeeming man from sin. He came to destroy all the works of the devil which try to stop us from living life to the fullness on earth. Therefore the works of Jesus also means to set us free from sickness and diseases.

"It is true that through the sin of one man death began to rule because of that one man. But how much greater is the result of what was done by the one man, Jesus Christ! All who receive God's abundant grace and are freely put right with him will rule in this life through Christ." (Romans 5:17) GNB.

Although we cannot see into the hearts of people who haven't been healed, I believe there are some factors we can look at to help us to maintain faith for our healing and for others that we pray for. While looking at some issues that prevented healing from taking place with great men or women of faith it will be helpful in seeing how these issues can also affect us. There are times when people are healed because of an atmosphere of healing that is in the place or building, and have nothing to do with the faith of the evangelist, minister or person who was praying for healing. God simply shows up and does what He does best.

At Bethel Church a popular saying is that "God likes to show up and show off." This isn't to slight or even suggest there was no faith on the part of the person who was ministering, but to simply reveal that God sometimes heals totally apart from faith or lack of faith on the part of the minister or even the people needing to be healed.

Some healing evangelists also operate in the gift of healing, gift of faith or gift of miracles as shown in 1 Corinthians 12. Even though these gifts may be in operation, it also may have nothing to do with the minister's personal faith. It's simply the Holy Spirit operating in what we call gifts of the Spirit operating through that minister.

"Now to each one the manifestation of the Spirit is given for the common good. To one there is given through the Spirit a message of wisdom, to another a message of knowledge by means of the same Spirit, to another faith by the same Spirit, to another gifts of healing by that one Spirit, to another miraculous powers, to another prophecy, to another distinguishing between spirits, to another speaking in different kinds of tongues, and to still another the interpretation of tongues. All these are the work of one and the same Spirit, and he distributes them to each one, just as he determines." (1Corinthians 12:7-11) NIV.

Ministers may not necessarily have personal faith for their own needs just because they are ministering out of the giftings of the Holy Spirit in meetings. God simply shows up through the Holy Spirit, and as a result, healings and miracles take place. With a gift in operation, people are healed through words of knowledge whereby the Holy Spirit, speaking through a person calls out a disease or sickness with the intent that God wants to heal a person from the sickness that was spoken.

Although many people are healed in meetings, many are also healed when ordinary people pray for them and lay hands on them.

*"These signs will follow those who believe: In My name they will cast out demons; they will speak with new tongues; they will take up serpents; and if they drink anything deadly, it will by no means hurt them; **they will lay hands on the sick, and they will recover**."* (my emphasis) *(Mark 16:17:18)* NKJV.

They can also be healed through anointing with oil and prayer.

*"Is anyone among you sick? Let him call for the elders of the church, and let them pray over him, anointing him with oil in the name of the Lord. And the **prayer of faith will save the sick, and the Lord will raise him up**. And if he has committed sins, he will be forgiven."* (my emphasis) *(James 5:14-15)* NKJV.

The point being emphasized is that healings and miracles can take place even if the person praying doesn't have faith for their own healing. Many have discovered that it's much easier to have faith for another person's healing than to have faith for their own healing.

There are many mysteries that will not be revealed this side of heaven, and I am certainly not attempting to point out any failures on the part of God's servants. There is no way I or anyone can know a leader's heart or personal faith level.

My only desire is to simply point out and defuse some things that the devil has used to destroy people's faith for healing as a result of leaders we had respected who died from diseases, especially if we're fighting the same disease. It's important that we don't allow satan to use the failures of others to weaken our own faith or destroy our belief in healing. We must stubbornly trust the veracity of God and His word, especially in the face of any failures or experiences of others or our present circumstances.

The present local pastor of Bethel Church is Bill Johnson's son, Eric Johnson. Eric was born with a major hearing deficiency. But because of his faith in God and the Bible, he never allows his own problems to hinder his belief that God has provided healing for everyone. Many deaf people have been instantly healed as he has prayed for them. He refuses to allow his faith to be affected by his own need of healing. Eric's faith rests only in what he believes in his heart about God and His word.

TRUE FAITH DOESN'T COME FROM WHAT WE SEE OR EXPERIENCE BUT FROM WHAT WE BELIEVE

In my fight against cancer, although I believed in healing, looking back, now recognize that the belief in my heart was different from what I believed in my head. As mentioned previously, it's far easier to pray for others in faith than to have faith for ourselves. And, like my experience, our lack of true heart faith is most often hidden from our own knowledge until something or Holy Spirit reveals it to us.

True faith is never determined only by what we say, what we see or by what we experience, but only what we believe in our hearts. If our faith is determined by what we experience or by the experiences of others, then our faith will go up or down according to those experiences. True faith is a product of authentic heart belief in God and His word.

Allow me to share an important thought for you to consider if you are contending against any attack from satan, no matter if it's spiritual, emotional or physical. We are all different, and all of us are at different places in operating in our faith and beliefs at any given time. Your situation doesn't hinder God from moving in your life. The good news is that He will always work with us in ways that are appropriate for us and for our particular situation.

During His time on earth, Jesus ministered to thousands of people who were obviously at different levels in their beliefs and levels of faith. And there were surely many who were in sin, yet the Bible says all who came to Him were healed.

"Jesus went about all of Galilee, teaching in their synagogues, preaching the gospel of the kingdom, and healing all kinds of sickness and all kinds of disease among the people. Then His fame went throughout all Syria; and they brought to Him all sick people

who were afflicted with various diseases and torments, and those who were demon-possessed, epileptics, and paralytics; and He healed them." (Matthew 4:23-24) NKJV.

The great truth is that Jesus hasn't changed, therefore He surely desires you to receive your healing. It doesn't matter what your condition, who you are, rich, poor, good or bad. The good news is that He has never changed. This very day, His healing is available for any and all who come to Him in faith. You can be healed today if you come to Him in faith. He hasn't changed!

GOD WILL ALWAYS PROVIDE EXACTLY WHAT WE NEED TO LIVE IN FAITH AND VICTORY

God will always provide exactly what you need to live in faith and victory according to your specific life and situation. With me it was necessary at that time in my life for God to come to me in a vision. I'm not totally sure why He came to me in that way. Perhaps it was because of what I had just gone through the previous year with my wife losing her battle with cancer. It may also have been necessary because God knew the specific tactics satan would be using against me. God never changes, but He does change His tactics and how He responds to our specific needs and situations in order to give us the best opportunity for victory.

YOU DON'T NEED GOD
TO COME IN A VISION
TO BE HEALED!!!

That is a vital truth. You don't need God to come to you in a vision in order to be healed. We make a grave mistake that puts us at a serious disadvantage if we decide or demand how God must operate in our lives. A vision was necessary for me, but isn't necessary for 99.9999 percent of people. It's enough for you to know that God is good and that He's on your side and has provided healing for you through the cross. He desires for you to receive the healing He paid for on the cross.

If you are contending against cancer or other major problems, I encourage you to look for your answer found in His words written to you in the Bible. His words of truth already have the answers to your problem. The major challenge for many of us is that we have difficulty believing that what He spoke in the Bible is for us personally, or we demand a multitude of passages before we will believe Him.

It's interesting that we often demand more of God than we do of people. We would probably lose many friends if we didn't trust the first words they spoke.

I recently had an experience that brings this home. A speaker at a church service made a simple statement that I hope many truly heard in their hearts. I know I understood and totally agreed with what she said. We must remember that it's what we hear and receive in our hearts that really matters. The speaker said some preachers use multitudes of passages in the Bible to prove a single point. Please understand that there is absolutely nothing wrong with a preacher using a multitude of passages to prove a point. What she was trying to say is that the problem stems or comes from the hearer's perspective.

She then went on to say that we would not need all those passages, if we would only believe the first passage. That spoke volumes because it reveals that all we need is to simply believe what God is saying to us the first time. If He only said it in one passage, that should be sufficient for us. Think about it, He didn't continually repeat the same thing in the Bible. He didn't give the 10 commandments to Moses twenty times. He had to rewrite them again because Moses broke the first stone tablets, but only spoke them one time.

Just think how foolish it would be if your wife had to tell you dinner was ready at least ten times in ten different ways. You wouldn't need her to say it a multitude of times or used a variety of words to convey that dinner was ready, especially if you were really hungry. It would be ridiculous if that were to happen. But how unreasonable is it to require God to tell us in multiple ways that He provided healing that is waiting for us to receive? Why should we demand more of God than we do from other people? We shouldn't need to have God repeat it over and over again in different ways before we believe and accept it.

If we require Him to speak a truth or promise over and over again, it reveals that we don't really believe that He or His word can be trusted. If you have a problem in trusting or believing the promises in the Bible, it would be a good time to ask Holy Spirit to reveal the cause of that unbelief.

We have found that often wounding from an earthly father or authority figure when young or even when older, affects in a negative way how we view or trust our heavenly father. It's amazing how healing from childhood wounds can improve faith and trust in God and His word.

Many times when we have been ministering to wounded hearts, people are healed physically without ever praying for healing, or they were healed without ever telling us they needed physical healing. Their emotional healing produced physical healing because they no longer feared God or believed He was rejecting them.

Failure to receive healing can also come as a result of wrong teaching, which produces a wrong belief and outlook concerning God and His desire to heal. The simple answer is to read and believe the truths found in the Bible through eyes that view God as good and One Who will do good for you.

Sometimes people may struggle with believing God will heal them because in their minds, they wrongly believe He has failed them in a past time of need. Some advocate that we should forgive God for failing us, but that's wrong theology and practice. Since God can't sin He couldn't have done anything wrong to require forgiveness.

Rather than forgive God, the proper response may be to repent for wrongly judging Him. However, before that can happen, the person needs to first ask the Holy Spirit to reveal the truth. Until the person understands that God didn't fail them, the pain and hurt will remain along with the inability to receive from Him. When Holy Spirit reveals truth the person will then be in a position to repent for wrongly judging God.

I earlier spoke of some of the ways people

are healed, such as through the operation of what is called the gifts of the Holy Spirit, anointing with oil or the laying on of hands. There are also times when people have been miraculously and instantly healed, but later lost their healing because there was no personal faith. Instead the healing was based on a gift in operation, another person's faith or the faith filled atmosphere in a place.

Any way you are healed is wonderful, but the greatest way is to be healed as a result of simply believing God's word. When you are healed because of your own faith in God's word, you won't lose your healing. Your confidence will be in God and His word, and not in another person's anointing or gifting. We would not need to go to healing meetings if we would simply believe God's Word.

*"By His stripes we **were** healed?"* (my emphasis). *(1 Peter 2:24)* NKJV.

The words "were healed" are written as past tense, not only because Jesus already paid the price for our sickness on the cross, but more important, is the truth that, in His eyes we are already healed.

"I am the Lord and I do not change." (Malachi 3:6) NKJV

Jesus was the very essence and express image of His Father as He lived and ministered to people. Over and over again in the gospels, it says He healed all who came to Him.   It's impossible for God to change His intent, desire or His ability! Jesus still wants to heal all who come to Him in faith just as He did when He was on earth. The following are a sampling of passages that reveal God's desire and will for you to be healed. I encourage you to read and meditate on these passages, and begin to read the Bible through eyes that see healing as a major desire and work of God, not just a side issue or something that only happened in history. The Bible is more than a history book. The Bible is a **His Story** and a **Your Story Book**. (Matthew 4:24, 8:16, 12:15, 14:14 & 36, 21:14; Mark 6:56; Luke 4:40, 6:17-19, 7:21-22, 9:11).

I encourage you to believe that God's Word

is still true today and that it is true for you. Read through all the healing accounts in the four Gospels and put yourself among the multitudes as they came to Jesus for healing. If your heart is open, you will come away healed because you are convinced that He still desires to heal everyone including you.

After many years of ministering healing to numerous people, there is no doubt that a major hindrance to healing is that many doubt it's God's will for them to be healed. I also believe the number one reason for this doubt is a result of wrong teaching from Bible teachers and preachers. I promise you that if you will set aside what you have been taught against healing and simply start believing what you're reading in the Bible, you will clearly see that healing is God's will for everyone including you. You can either believe a man who is fallible or believe God who is not only infallible, but is also a God Who cannot and will never lie. Your choice!

Jesus was the express will of God on earth, and His actions of healing everyone who came to Him should be evidence enough for anyone who has an open mind to see that God still desires for everyone to be healed who come to Him.

EVERYONE IS WORTHY TO RECEIVE HEALING, NOT JUST A CHOSEN FEW

Unworthiness seems to be a major hindrance to people receiving healing in spite of the fact that the Bible clearly reveals we have all been made worthy through Jesus. The truth is that the Bible clearly teaches that all believers in Jesus Christ, individually and corporately not only make up the body of Christ, but in that truth we are assured that everyone is worthy to receive healing, not just a chosen few.

Jesus is the head, and we are His body, loved by all of the Godhead. And I might add that it was God's idea and choice to have us become the body of Christ while we were still sinners.

"God has put all things under the authority of Christ and has made Him head over all things for the benefit of the church. And the church

is **His body**; it is made full and complete by Christ, who fills all things everywhere with Himself." (my emphasis) *(Ephesians 1:22-23)* NLT.

"Now these are the gifts Christ gave to the church: apostles, prophets, evangelists, the pastors and teachers. Their responsibility is to equip God's people to do His work and build up the church, the **body of Christ**. (my emphasis) *(Ephesians 4:12-13)* NLT (See also 1 Corinthians 12:12-27, Colossians 2:9-10).

I would like to illustrate how beloved you are by Jesus, Holy Spirit and the Father, and how much They desire to care for you and see you healed. Imagine that you are in the hospital emergency room with two broken arms when a doctor comes and begins to work on your right arm. You immediately stop him and tell him to only fix your left arm. He is perplexed because he knows full well that both arms are broken and need attention, and that his calling in life is to help people in need. He wants to help you, but you stop him from doing what he desires to do.

He is obviously confused as to why you won't allow him to work on your right arm, so he questions your reasoning. So you say, "doctor, with this arm I wrote checks when I knew I didn't have money in the bank. With this arm I signed my tax forms knowing that I had lied about my income and deductions. With this arm I abused my wife and children. With this arm I did some things that were very terrible. This arm doesn't deserve to be healed and made well."

You would never stop a doctor from helping you! You would want the doctor to do everything he could possibly do to stop the pain and bring healing to both of your arms. You would want the doctor's help because you love your whole body no matter how that part acted, or what that part was responsible for. The love Jesus has for His body is far greater than any love we could have for our own bodies. If we love our bodies enough to want every part well and healthy, just imagine how much more Jesus loves every part of His body, and wants every part of His body well and healthy, no matter what you have done or how you have acted!

I would like to paint another picture for you in order to help you understand how much God loves you and desires to see you healed. Almost all Bible scholars believe that we're a spirit being who is the real person, and that we have or possess a soul which is our mind, will and emotions, and we live in a house called our bodies.

Picture a glass with some water in it. The glass is your body and the water is your spirit who is the real you. There is another glass of water, which represents the Godhead. If you were to take the glass containing the Godhead and pour the water into your glass it would mix with your water and become one water. The Bible clearly teaches that when we are born again, the Godhead is in us and we are in the Godhead.

*"At that day you will know that I am in My Father, and **you in Me, and I in you.**"*(my emphasis) *(John 14:20)* NKJV.

"Christ in you, is the hope of glory. (my

emphasis) *(Colossians 1:27)* NKJV.

"Do you not know that you are the temple of God and that the Spirit of God **dwells in you**?"(my emphasis) *(1Corinthians 3:16)* NKJV.

"For we are the temple of the living God. As God has said: **"I will live in them** *and walk among them, and I will be their God, and they will be my people."* (my emphasis) *(2Corinthians 6:16)* NKJV.

I encourage you to read Romans 6, Ephesians and Colossians, noting how many times the Bible speaks of us being in Jesus and the Godhead in us. We are truly one in spirit with God. We aren't Gods, but when we become believers, we have the same essence as God and are one with the Godhead. The entire Godhead lives in us through the indwelling of the Holy Spirit. This happens the moment that we are born again, or more accurately born from above, becoming what we call Believers or Christians.

"Anyone united to the Lord becomes **one spirit with him**." (my emphasis) *(1Corinthians*

6:17) NIV.

To help us better understand this passage, and what the Bible is speaking about us being in the Godhead and the Godhead being in us, imagine pouring cream, which represents the Godhead, into a cup of coffee which represents us. The coffee is still coffee and the cream is still cream, but they are now inseparable. We will never become God, but we are forever united with the Godhead. Another way to look at it is to imagine looking at an ocean, and in every direction you look, all you can see is water. You see a drop of water fall into the ocean, and realize that drop became part of the ocean. It doesn't become the ocean, but becomes a part of it, and can never be separated from it. The ocean is God and you are the drop. You will never be God, but you are forever a part of Him and can never be separated from Him.

Since the passage in First Corinthians says we are now one spirit with Him, it would be impossible for God to not love you. It would be impossible for God to not want to protect you. It would be impossible for

God to not want to provide for you. And, it would be impossible for God to not want you healed. God is now part of you and you are now part of God. For God to do less would be to say that if it were possible for Him to have a broken arm, He wouldn't want it healed. God is not against Himself or His body. Settle it in your heart. You are part of His body and He loves every part of His body. God wants everyone healed and He wants **you** healed!

I want to make something perfectly clear to any non-believers reading this book. I want you to understand that when Jesus went to the cross He provided healing for everyone, including non-believers. God loves you as much as the most devoted believer and desires you to be healed! And, He won't make you jump through any hoops in order to be healed! He will heal you because He is a caring and compassionate God. He loves to heal and do good things for us, not because of our actions, our lifestyles, or who we are, but because of Who He is.

The Bible is very clear in showing that Jesus healed everyone who came to Him, without ever asking them if they wanted to become His follower or not. And that was during a period of time when everyone He came in contact with was still living under the law, before He ever went to the cross to bring redemption.

Jesus did far more than redeem us from our sin. The cross was a complete work of God through Jesus which provided total healing of our entire being, of our spirits, souls and bodies. The Bible says that God loved and still loves the whole world so much that He sent His Son Jesus to redeem everyone.

God never stops loving anyone, irregardless of their life style or actions. Many who have a ministry of praying for people to be healed, will admit that it's sometimes easier for a nonbeliever to be healed than for a believer. We will explain the reasons for this seeming paradox further on. I encourage you to begin declaring that healing is for you. In the book of Job there is a great truth and promise for us.

"You will declare **a thing** (my emphasis) *and it will be established for you and light will*

shine on your ways." (Job 22:28). NKJV.

The word "thing" is a poor translation of the Hebrew word. In the original language it carries a meaning of a command, promise or a word from God. It's error and foolish to think we can declare anything we want out of lust or selfishness, and then expect it to be established. But, we do have full authority and every right to declare a command, a word or promise from God and His Word. When we do, there is an assured expectation that it will be established in our lives.

The word "declare" is a judicial term that carries the weight and authority of heaven, which is far greater than when an earthly judge declares that a person is either guilty or innocent. If a judge's declaration carries the authority of the earthly court system, how much more do our declarations carry the weight and authority of God's heavenly court system. The Bible reveals that we are seated in the heavenly realm in Jesus, and that the entire Godhead is on our side. We are the family of God and the body of Christ. Our loving heavenly Father will surely take care of His children, as surely as Christ will take care of His body.

We can be assured that when we declare a command or promise of God, it not only carries the weight and authority of heaven's court, but God's ministering spirits will work on our behalf to make sure that what we declare will be established in our lives, and the light of God will shine upon it.

"Are not all angels ministering spirits sent to serve those who will inherit salvation?" (Hebrews 1:14) NIV.

A parting word on this thought is an exhortation for you to find the truths and promises from God's Word, and then begin to declare them over your life until they reside in your heart and manifest in your life. When your heart and your words come into agreement with God's promises, they will absolutely be established in your life.

"I will not die but live, and will proclaim what the Lord has done." Psalms 118:17 NKJV.

This is a great example and promise for anyone. It's impossible for nothing to happen when we pray. Something always happens. We may not see it instantly in the physical realm, but it has happened in God's invisible realm the moment we pray.

If we aren't going to believe His Word on healing if it isn't instantly manifested, what is the basis for believing in heaven or our salvation? The reality of heaven isn't personally manifested yet either, so what is the difference? The difference is we believe God's word on salvation, but not healing because the devil does everything he can to stop us from experiencing God's abundant life on earth which He purchased for us on the cross.

It's vital that we live by His Word, not by sight and thank Him for healing us even if it seems nothing has happened. Thanksgiving will always produce results. True thanksgiving never focuses on what hasn't happened, but on what He has done according to His word as though it were completely finished.

*"By His stripes we **were healed.** (my emphasis). (1 Peter 2:24)* NKJV.

QUANTUM PHYSICS AND HEALING

I would like to briefly delve into Quantum physics because it can be a tremendous faith builder as well as a tool to assist you in receiving healing or healing for others, when you pray for them.

In Quantum physics, a quark is an elementary particle and a fundamental constituent of matter. Quarks combine to form composite particles called hadrons, the most stable of which are photons, protons and neutrons, the components of atomic nuclei. In the study of Quantum physics, something takes place that not only mystifies physicists, but also goes against all logical thinking and what is considered normal physics. Without going into all the experiments and tests, the following results, although overly simplified, is what they discovered through numerous experiments by multitudes of men and women.

When they observe the tiny particles of an atom, the particles would behave in such a way as to become what the observer expected to see. They would try to trick the particles without success. The particles seemed to know ahead of time what the people expected to see and took on that very form.

Everything from the chairs we sit on, our cars, or cell phones are made up of atoms. Everything in our universe is comprised of atoms which includes everything in the visible and invisible realms. As a matter of fact, it's generally understood that we only see about seven percent of reality, while 93 percent of reality is in the invisible realm. More important, we as human beings are made up of atoms including not just our bodies, but also our invisible souls and spirits. I hope you can grasp the ramifications and where this is going. Because we are composed of atoms, whatever we expect to see has the potential to become what we are expecting, either for good or bad.

WHAT WE EXPECT TO SEE HAS THE POTENTIAL TO PRODUCE THE EXPECTED RESULTS

Concerning sickness and our bodies, there is a potential for the atoms to become more firmly engrained as a disease or sickness, or the potential to become healthy atoms which in turn produce healthy cells and organs in our bodies. Because we are made up of atom particles, they can become what we are expecting or believing for, just as all the physicists discovered in their experiments.

"If we believe in our hearts and confess with our mouth, salvation (healing) *comes."* (my insert). *(Roman's 10:10)* NKJV.

As I thought of this in the context of quantum physics I realized the potential positive impact we can have when praying for ourselves or others. As mentioned earlier, the meaning of the word used for salvation is sozo, which includes deliverance, protection, provision, **and healing**. It is better understood to be an all-inclusive term that means to fix whatever is broken and restore all that is missing.

"Truly I tell you, if anyone says to this mountain, Go, throw yourself into the sea and does not doubt in their heart but believes that what they say (expect) *will happen, it will be done for them. Therefore I tell you, whatever you ask for in prayer, believe that you have received it, and it will be yours."* (my insert) *(Mark 11:23-24)* NRSV.

If we truly believe in our heart (or expect) what we are praying for, the Bible says that we already have it. It may still be in the invisible realm, but if we don't waiver in our faith and hold onto our confession of that truth, we will see it manifested in the natural realm. It may not be instant, but it will come.

"Let us not grow weary in doing good, for at the proper time we will reap, if we do not give up." (Galatians 6:9) LEB.

"Let us hold tightly without wavering to the hope we affirm (or believe what we have), *for*

God can be trusted to keep His promise." (my insert), *(Hebrews 10:13)* NLT.

As we pray for the sick, and believe and see in our hearts and imaginations that all the cancer cells are being restored to healthy cells, then because our bodies are made up of atoms, what we are expecting to occur, has the potential to be empowered to happen. All the atoms which make up our body cells have the potential to be reformed into what we expect to see (believe or have faith for), either for good or bad. The atoms in our bodies have the potential to react, just like what the physicists discovered in their experiments and tests.

Although the majority of the medical world has no grid for faith healing or for quantum physics in relation to healing, they do have a grid for positive thinking. Many hospitals in dealing with patients who have major medial diseases or illnesses, have found positive results in having patients attempt to see and imagine themselves well and doing things they couldn't do unless they were healed. The medical world unknowingly agree with Solomon when he said that what we speak can either produce life or death.

Medical science has also proven that depending on what we speak, our brains will release chemicals that will cause our bodies to either be energized or slow down. Kinesiology muscle testing also reveals that when we speak negative words or even think negative thoughts, our muscles become weak, but will have strength when we think positive thoughts or speak positive words.

Isn't it amazing that it has taken medicine and science over 3,000 years to catch up to what God spoke through Solomon. It has been medically proven that our bodies can even kill pain by releasing endorphins if we speak life instead of death over ourselves.

When ministering physically healing to people, we will often have them talk to their bodies, and they are amazed when pain and other symptoms disappear.

Here is a thought for us to consider. We can align our words and thoughts with the Word of God and use our authority in Jesus or use chemicals and drugs to make the medical industry rich and ourselves poor. If I am going to become an addict, I choose to become addicted to Jesus and His power, and not prescription drugs.

In reality there isn't much difference between prescription pain drugs and street drugs in respect to becoming addicted. There are only two major differences between street drugs and prescription drugs. Prescription pain drugs are legal and Street drugs illegal. The other main difference is prescription pain drugs are exorbitant in price while street drugs are relatively cheap. The other fact is that many times prescription pain drugs especially those containing fentanyl lead to using street drugs.

Please understand that unlike the experiments in Quantum Physics, in our expectations of physical healing for others, we must always factor in a person's free will and their faith, when praying for them. God created us with free wills and will not violate anyone's will.

"You are free to eat from any tree in the garden. But you must never eat from the tree of the knowledge of good and evil because when you eat from it, you will certainly die." (Genesis 2:16-17)

In essence God said the day you choose or exercise your free will to eat of the wrong tree you will die. This is a much debated area, for some have experienced what appeared to be times when healing or other things took place that appeared to go against a person's will. Often it isn't that they were against being healed, but were healed because of your faith which produced their healing in spite of their lack of faith. Unlike God, we don't know what's in a person's heart no matter what they speak or what their actions may be. There are also some mysteries we will never have answers for this side of heaven.

All we can do is refer back to the Word of God. The Bible teaches us that God created man with a free will to choose good or evil. God didn't desire Adam and Eve to choose to eat of the forbidden tree. But, God on purpose wanted man to choose Him of their own free will.

Without free will, God would be unjust to punish us for sinful things we did against our will. We can always choose good or evil, or choose to believe or not believe, no matter what others expect of us.

In ministering healing to others, there is also a great possibility that there may be situations or things going on in their life that may hinder them from receiving healing. In those situations, we must rely on the Holy Spirit to reveal what that may be and how He would want us to deal with the issues. This also applies to our own lives when the manifestation of healing doesn't come or is delayed.

It is important for us to understand that our faith and beliefs which can be equated to our expectations have the potential to alter the very atoms which make up our physical bodies. Our expectations have the ability to cause the atoms in our bodies to change from damaged or cancerous cells to become healthy cells. This means we must be very careful to make sure that our expectations line up with God's word, His nature and His character.

Another connection between Quantum physics and healing is what is known as quantum entanglement. What they discovered in their experiments was that whenever a particle, a photon in the tests, acted in a certain way, the partner photon acted the same. In the experiments, they managed to divide a photon, and then changed the spin direction of one of them, and to their surprise, the other photon also changed its spin direction. They found that it didn't matter if the divided photons were two feet apart or across the galaxy, they always acted in unison. This phenomenon has been repeated again and again with the same results, along with photographs as further proof. It may not seem important on the surface, but has everything to do with not only healing, but all facets of our life.

"as He is, so are we in this world." (1 John 4:17) NKJV

Although the passage is specifically

referring to love in the chapter, the overriding truth and principles apply to all areas of our life. Jesus lives in heaven today with a physical body which He demonstrated when He ate with His disciples after His resurrection.

"Do you have anything here to eat?" They gave him a piece of broiled fish, and He took it and ate it in their presence. (Luke 24:42-43) NKJV

The Bible clearly teaches that He is in us and we are in Him through the Holy Spirit, and also teaches us that He is our head and we are His body. We are totally connected just like the photons in Quantum Entanglement. That is why Jesus could say as He is in heaven, so we are in this world.

When it comes to healing, Jesus is perfectly healthy, which means since He is healthy in heaven, which means in His eyes we are healthy in our earthly world. As we believe and declare this truth, it will become manifested in us on earth.

PRAYING FOR OTHERS

I would like to address how we pray for ourselves or others. Too often we have a tendency to say long prayers. Long prayers are often an indication of wrong beliefs and lack of faith.

With long prayers we're often trying to convince ourselves that God wants to heal us or another person. Long prayers often mean we're trying to convince God to do what we want. When we attempt to persuade God to do something we don't think He wants to do, we're practicing witchcraft by trying to control or manipulate Him. We don't need to convince God to do what He already has provided for us on the cross. When we have the correct beliefs in our hearts and pray in faith, we'll discover that simple childlike prayers will move mountains.

This seems like a great opportunity to kick over a sacred cow and risk making some people angry. Please don't gather wood and matches to burn me at the stake but, it's unbiblical to ask God to heal us! As far as He's concerned, He has already healed us through Jesus.

"These signs will follow those who believe: In My name they will cast out demons; they will speak with new tongues; they will take up serpents; and if they drink anything deadly, it will by no means hurt them; they will lay hands on the sick, and they will recover." (Mark 16:17-18) NKJV

Many people ignore or repudiate this account because they get all hung up on the serpent handling and drinking poison aspect of this passage. The bible is full of metaphors and figurative language. Jesus is no more talking about literal serpents or poison in this verse than He was saying Herod was a literal fox.

"Go tell that fox that I will keep on casting out demons and healing people today and tomorrow; and the third day I will accomplish My purpose." (Luke 13:32) NLT

Jesus is telling us through figurative

language that we don't have to fear the devil and his minions (serpents) because we have power and authority over them. And the poison refers to poisonous words and verbal attacks we will encounter, but not to be concerned because we won't be harmed by them. The snake handler churches have taken this passage literally to their harm, and also caused harm to the testimony of the church. Although Jesus is using figurative language, there have also been numerous testimonies of God preventing harm to people who have been bitten by venomous snakes or by drinking poison, as seen in Acts 28, when the Apostle Paul was not harmed after being bitten by a poisonous snake.

In this passage in Mark, "they will lay hands on the sick, and they will recover," Jesus says nothing about praying and asking God to heal the person. In the midst of revealing what His Father was like as He healed and performed many miracles, He was also training His followers and modeling how they were to minister to people. There is no mention of Jesus asking God to heal anyone. Jesus simply commanded demons to leave and healed the people with a word.

Unspoken in this passage is that He expected us to do as He did. He commissioned His 12 apostles and later the 70 disciples, and gave them (and us) power and authority, and simply told them to heal the sick and cast out demons, not too beg or even ask God to heal them. And, that was even before the cross!

In the Old Testament, it was proper to ask God to heal people because Jesus hadn't yet gone to the cross. The purpose of the cross was much more than paying for our sins so we could go to heaven. The work of the cross was a complete work that was meant to redeem spirit, soul and body. (See Isaiah 53:4-5, Matthew 8:16-17, 1Peter 2:24)

I would like you to consider who we are as children of God and believers in Jesus Christ. Jesus is the head and we are His body. Should not the body do what and how the head would do?

It is our responsibility to receive the healing that was already made available on the cross, and to lay hands on others to be healed as we see with Peter and John with the crippled man at the gate beautiful.

"In the name of Jesus Christ of Nazareth, rise up and walk." (Acts 3:6) NKJV

Peter didn't say, "let me pray and ask God and see if He is willing to heal you," nor did he beg God to heal the man. He simply operated in his authority as a believer in Jesus Christ and the man was healed. The apostle Paul did the same in Acts 14:10, and Peter again in Acts 9:34 and Acts 9:40.

They both simply ministered as Jesus would have done. As believers we're to do the same and command people to be healed in the name that is above every name. We are to speak to the disease, sickness or pain and command it to leave in the mighty name of Jesus. We're to call forth and release healing and even recreation of body parts, new hearts, new eyes, new lungs, and kidneys, not to mention we are to speak to dead bodies and call them back to life in the name and authority of Jesus Christ. We're to command the body parts to work according to God's design.

And, when Holy Spirit reveals the source is demonic, we're to command the spirits out. We're to command deaf and dumb spirits, epileptic spirits, blind spirits, ALS spirits to come out in the name of Jesus Christ, because His Name is above every name in the heavens and on earth.

Angels are here to assist us, but Jesus didn't say we're to call angels to do what He called us to do. We are to cast out demons and lay hands on the sick and then watch God do His work to validate His Word. God gave us authority to live out His word and act on it. As we act, angels will assist us, but they won't do what we're called to do.

Jesus also never said long prayers. He simply said, "be healed," or "stretch out your hand." When He cast out demons, He simply said "come out."

Receiving or ministering healing has nothing to do with how well or long we pray, but does have everything to do with knowing God's will to heal, and knowing our authority and the power that resides in the name of Jesus. Peter gave the perfect answer to how the crippled man at the Gate Beautiful was healed.

"By faith in the name of Jesus, this man whom you see and know was made strong. It is Jesus' name and the faith that comes through him that has completely healed him, as you can all see." (Acts 3:16) NIV.

When we know in our hearts, the authority we have as believers, and truly believe that God is good and that He desires everyone to be healed we'll find long prayers aren't necessary.

Remember the often used WWJD phrase of a few years ago? Perhaps we should utilize a "HWJP" phrase. Before praying for people, it may be good to ask ourselves, "How Would Jesus Pray?" Keeping it simple could very well bring the same results that Jesus had. It's **our faith in God and His Word,** and not faith is the specific words or prayers which will produce healing.

Another aspect of how Jesus prayed is often the opposite of how we pray. Jesus never begged God to heal the person, nor did

He try to convince God to heal the person because they were a good person and deserved to be healed, like a lot prayers I have heard people pray. Because Jesus knew God's will, He simply commanded healing to come or demons to leave. Jesus knew God's will for healing, and therefore knew God would back Him up. God is the healer, but we're His representatives on earth.

If you are reading this book in the midst of contending against a sickness or disease, I encourage you to stop reading and speak aloud the following prayer over yourself and receive it into your heart.

*In the name of Jesus Christ, I command this (name the sickness problem) to leave me now. The Word of God in First Peter 2:24 says, "by His stripes we **were** healed." That means I am already healed. Therefore I declare I will rise up totally healed and free of all symptoms. I will hold fast to the Word of God until my healing is totally manifested. I declare I am full of the joy of the lord and I will live out my life totally free of pain and sickness. I declare when it comes time for me to go home to Jesus, I will be like Moses, and leave this earthly* *world full of strength, life and vitality. Thank you Jesus, I am healed in Your Name which is above (name the sickness or problem). Amen!*

SATAN ISN'T THE ONLY HINDRANCE TO RECEIVING YOUR HEALING

I would like to briefly mention some things that hinder us from receiving healing, because satan isn't the only direct hindrance to people being healed. I have already addressed some and will cover the others more thoroughly, but feel it's good to place them in a list as a reminder.

Guilt and condemnation from sin, (especially unforgiveness in believers). In depth coverage will follow.

We aren't always totally convinced that God is good or that it's His will to heal everyone all the time. Many actually believe and many preachers even teach from the pulpits that God makes us sick. We need to stop believing the devil's lie that every time something bad happens, that God is punishing us or teaching us a lesson. Just because sickness and pain gets our attention, and as a result God produces something good out of it, doesn't mean He's behind what happened. God isn't the author of pain and sickness, but He really does a fantastic job of making lemonade out of lemons.

"We can glory in our tribulations (our lemons), *because we know that tribulations* (our Lemons) *produces perseverance* (while the lemonade is being made)*; and our perseverance produces approved character; and our approved character produces hope. And hope does not disappoint us, because God's love has been poured out into our hearts through the Holy Spirit, who has been given to us."* (my inserts) *(Romans 5:3-5)* ISV

It's safe to say that Paul had his share of tests and trials. Speaking out his own experiences he was able to address God's ability to take the evil the enemy does and give us victories in the midst of troubles.

*"We know that **in everything** God works for the good of those who love Him."* (my emphasis) *(Romans 8:28)* ERV

"God is good and only does good" (Psalm

119:68) NKJV

If we can ever get it in our spirit that God is good and only does good, and that He truly and deeply loves us unconditionally, we would never accept the devil's lie that God is the one who is behind all the destructive things that happen in the world or to us.

The very word "unconditional love," means it has absolutely nothing to do with how we think or act, nor does it have anything to do with whether we love Him back, ignore Him or actively fight against Him.

Love is Who God is, and because His very nature is love, that which flows out of Him is love towards all of mankind. Just as water naturally flows from a water spring without outside action, unconditional love naturally flows from our loving heavenly Father without outside action.

No decent earthly father who lives in a sinful world, and who is constantly bombarded and tempted to sin, would ever make his child sick to teach him a lesson or punish him with a deadly disease. How sad and wretched that we would ever even consider it would be possible for a loving Father Who sacrificed His Son for us would ever stoop to such despicable actions.

The only thing a judge could ever convict God for is that He oozes love and compassion for all of His creation. Instead of blaming God for everything, we need to understand there are many other factors at work in our world to produce sickness or diseases. We live in a sinful world, where the majority are non-believers who are capable of hurting and destroying others on purpose.

Sinful people, because of greed, contaminate air, water and food sources which often becomes an open door through which our enemy works to bring sickness, disease and death. We live in a fallen world full of germs, disease, drugs and sinful people. It's no wonder the devil has an easy time to create pain, injuries, sickness, disease and premature death. God wasn't the one who listened to the devil and ate the forbidden fruit which brought sin into the world and into mankind.

God created mankind with a free will, and that includes people who intentionally hurt others, or spread diseases like HIV or Aids. God isn't responsible for the sinful use of our free will.

Before we throw stones at God, perhaps it would be good to ask ourselves if we have ever used our free will wrongly and caused harm to others, and if so, was God the guilty one or us?

It's only because of God's grace that we don't suffer more than we deserve.

Every decent parent knows that their responsibility is to provide protection, comfort, provision and direction for their children, and to care for them in every area of need. Do we honestly believe that our Heavenly Father would do less for us than imperfect earthly parents? It doesn't make sense that Jesus would die for the cause and root of all sickness, which is sin, and not take care of the results. That is like cleaning all the glass and nails from the road, but not fixing the flat tire.

As stated earlier; I absolutely agree with

people who say the day of miracles is past, because there never was a day or season of miracles, only a God of miracles. However, He is God Who has never changed, and therefore will heal in all dispensations or times. It's ridiculous to think He's good one day or time, and not good at other times. That is like a child's mother saying she will only feed him on Sundays, Mondays and Fridays, but not to expect her to feed him or her the other days.

Not believing you are healed unless you see instant change. Faith or belief must come before, not just after we have received the possession or manifestation of healing. Bible faith sees the future as past tense action. I will address this in great depth further on.

Believing you must be good enough for God to heal you. There's no perfect person on earth, nor is there a measuring point we must reach or attain to receive healing. It's God's goodness that heals us, not who we are or what we have done, either good or bad.

Making man's medicine plan A, and only seeking God as a back-up policy if man's way does not work. That's not faith, but desperation. I covered this earlier, but would like to mention a few additional thoughts. There is nothing wrong with going to doctors, provided our faith is in God first and foremost, and not in man. There should be first and foremost God as plan A, and utilizing doctors working in conjunction with God, not as a replacement for Him.

The devil is not ignorant or stupid, but is very wise and sly. His wisdom is very twisted because of his sin, but we must never underestimate his ability or his tactics.

Something that has crept in very strongly is in the area of supplements. It's not that supplements are evil. It's not that we're in sin or making a mistake if we're taking them. They can be beneficial, especially as we age in order to make up for the necessary vitamins and minerals that are lacking in many foods because of depleted nutrients in our soils. The challenge is the same as making doctors and medical procedures our plan A. What are you placing your faith in? God or supplements?

The question we must ask ourselves is, will taking supplements cause us to compromise our faith in God's provision? We must always be careful to not allow our faith in God to be misplaced by faith in natural supplements, even though they are for the most part beneficial and less dangerous to us than prescription drugs.

The other aspect to consider is to determine where your level of faith is concerning your belief in God's provision. We should be very careful about urging anyone to stop taking prescription drugs or supplements and just trust God. That must always be the person's decision because only they truly know their level of belief and faith.

The devil would love to destroy a person with wrong decisions when they are contending against a disease or sickness. The best advice is to encourage the person to seek discernment from Holy Spirit in how they should contend for their healing and health. There is no "fits all" size for healing.

UNFORGIVENESS CAN STOP US FROM RECEIVING HEALING

An important topic that needs to be addressed is the impact that unforgiveness plays in regards to whether people are able to receive healing. We have found in ministering healing to numerous people that there are many times when unforgiveness may prevent people from receiving their healing. Please understand that God desires to heal everyone, and sin of any type, in and of itself will never change God's desire to heal you. All one has to do, is read the four gospels to see that Jesus never laid any requirements on people other than faith. And, there were many times when it seems that He healed people even when they didn't appear to have faith. God is truly good all the time, and is only capable of doing what is good.

Sin in their life also never appeared to stop Jesus from healing people. The Bible says that He healed everyone who came to Him.

In the Gospel of John we see that Jesus healed the cripple at the pool of Bethesda, and only later did He tell him to stop his sinning.

"Later Jesus found him at the temple and said to him, See, you are well again. Stop sinning or something worse may happen to you." (John 5:14) NIV

The important truth is that the man's sin didn't stop Jesus from healing him. In Luke after the cripple was let down through the roof, Jesus said, *"your sins are forgiven you." (Luke 5:20)*. NIV.

The man obviously had sin in his life which prompted Jesus to forgive him. I add that the man never even asked Jesus to forgive him. But the main point is that it didn't stop Jesus from wanting to heal him. True to their colors, the Scribes and Pharisees quickly complained that only God can forgive sins prompting Jesus to respond.

"That you may know the Son of Man has power on earth to forgive sins, He said to the man who was paralyzed, I say to you take up your bed and walk and go to your

house." (Luke 5:24) NIV

All four gospels tell of multitudes coming to be healed, and that Jesus healed all who came to Him. Among all the multitudes, you can be sure there was sin in many of them. But Jesus never refused to heal anyone or place any preconditions on them before He healed them. Some have found there are times when it is easier for non-Christians to be healed than Christians. Miracles and healings are signs and wonders which point to something, just as signs point to the way into a building or road signs lead us to destinations. When non-believers are healed and experience God's love for them, they often give their lives to Him.

By saying this, I'm not condoning sin, but merely stating that God is a loving Father Who delights in drawing people to Himself through healings and miracles. God is far bigger than our sin, which is great news because the only human who was totally free of sin was Jesus.

"If you sin, how does that affect God? If your

sins are many, what does that do to Him? If you are righteous, what do you give to Him, or what does He receive from your hand? Your wickedness only affects humans like yourself, and your righteousness only affects other people." (Job 35:6-8) NIV.

Our righteousness doesn't make God look or become any better, any more than our sins will make Him look or become any worse. In the Old Testament, touching a leper could not only infect you with their leprosy, but you were considered unclean if you did touch one.

Although the four Gospels are found in the New Testament section of our Bibles, except for the last chapters in each book, it was still life under the Old Testament law. In touching the leper, Jesus not only revealed His identity as God by making the man clean instead of Himself being made unclean, but also demonstrated that He was greater than sin or disease.

Not to contradict myself, sin can sometimes appear to hinder people from receiving healing, especially with

Christians, however it isn't the sin itself that hinders, but the resulting guilt and self-condemnation of that sin. The following passage gives us some insight into how we may be hindered from being healed or from receiving answers to prayer.

*"Little children, let us not love in word or talk but in deed and in truth. By this we shall know that we are of the truth and reassure our heart before him; for whenever **our heart condemns us**, God is greater than our heart, and he knows everything. Beloved, if our heart does not condemn us, we have confidence before God; and whatever we ask we receive from him, because we keep his commandments and do what pleases him."* (my emphasis) *(1John 3:18-23).* NKJV.

It is important to note that this passage reveals that it isn't God who is condemning us. He came to save us, not condemn us. It's our own heart which is condemning us, because deep down we know that our actions are wrong.

Our faith goes out the window if consciously or sub-consciously our heart condemns us. There are times people have been healed because of the faith of the minister or because of the anointing that is in the atmosphere, but they sometimes lose their healing. One reason is because of self-condemnation, shame and guilt, which gives the enemy an open door to attack them again with the same illness. That was the likely outcome with the crippled man that Jesus healed at the pool of Bethesda.

"Afterward Jesus found him in the Temple and told him, "Now you are well; so stop sinning, or something even worse may happen to you." (John 5:14)

The man was healed because of the faith of Jesus, not his own faith, and it appears that Jesus knew his sin would open the door for satan to bring guilt and self-condemnation and cause him to lose his healing, so He told him to stop his sinning.

What we have discovered and proven after ministering to countless people over many years, is that un-forgiveness is the sin which causes the most problems, and it seems to be predominately among

Believers. One reason is that because deep in a believer's heart, he or she knows that God commands them to not hold offenses, but to forgive others.

It's sometimes easier for unbelievers to receive healing because they aren't affected nearly as much by guilt and condemnation of sin or in this case a result of holding unforgiveness against someone. I suspect it's because they are either unaware what God says about it or they simply don't care what He thinks.

When I was an unbeliever, sin was no big deal to me. My thinking at the times was, "hey, I am just as good or even better than a lot of people I know, but if I end up in hell at least I will be with all my friends." Pretty stupid isn't it, but that is the sentiment of many unbelievers.

Preachers often use Habakkuk to say God can't look on sin because He's too holy, as a way to legalistically bring guilt and condemnation to get their people to stop sinning and do what is right.

"Your eyes are too pure to look at what is evil.

You can't put up with the wrong things people do. So why do You put up with those who can't be trusted?" (Habakkuk 1:13) NIRV

The problem is that they only use the first part of the verse. The Prophet was really saying that a holy God should not have to look at sin. In the second part of the passage he then asked, so why do you look at their sin? Try telling Adam, Cain or all the people before the flood or Sodom and Gomorrah that God can't see or look at sin.

There have been times when I would have preferred that God didn't see or look at my sin. But, the truth is that God not only sees outward sin, but as the Bible says, He sees everything in our hearts, including our sinful thoughts and sinful motives.

Good News! God isn't fazed by our sin. I'm not in any way condoning sin, but God is so much bigger than our sin, and His love extends far beyond our actions.

A major reason we often find it hard to forgive someone is because of the deep wounds they have caused. These deep heart wounds often result in resentment, bitterness, thoughts of revenge, anger, and other negative thoughts or actions.

*"If you forgive other people when they sin against you, your heavenly Father will also forgive you. But if you do not forgive others their sins, your Father **will not forgive your sins.**"* (my emphasis) *(Matthew 6:14-15)* NIV.

That sounds pretty scary, dogmatic and seems to indicate an angry God, but Mark's account gives us more clarity in what God desires us to understand.

"Truly I tell you, if anyone says to this mountain, Go, throw yourself into the sea, and does not doubt in their heart but believes that what they say will happen, it will be done for them. Therefore I tell you, whatever you ask for in prayer, believe that you have received it, and it will be yours. And when you stand praying, (seeking to be healed) *if you hold anything against anyone, forgive them, so that your Father in heaven **may forgive you your sins**.* (my insert and emphasis). *(Mark 11:23-25)* NIV.

The key words are "may forgive you your

sins." This is a supporting thought to what we found in the 1 John 3:18-23 passage about our own heart condemning us.

In Mark's account, we can surmise that when we hold unforgiveness against someone, consciously or sub-consciously, we'll feel condemned in our hearts and won't be able to receive God's forgiveness. It isn't that God is unwilling to forgive us, but that we aren't able to receive His forgiveness because of self-condemnation and guilt. We can believe with our heads that He has forgiven us, and even speak that He has, but deep in our hearts we'll feel condemned and won't be able to truly receive His forgiveness if we haven't forgiven others.

And if we're not able to receive His forgiveness, we won't have confidence or faith that God will hear or answer our prayer to be healed, as shown in the 1 John 3:18-23 passage.

The guilt and condemnation comes because deep in our hearts we know we shouldn't hold un-forgiveness. We either refuse because we want them to pay for what they did to us or we don't know how to fully forgive others.

From too many pulpits God is labeled as some hard-nosed dictator. They declare that God is always watching and waiting to catch us in some sin, and when that happens He will punish us or withhold His favor and blessings from us.

We're in major trouble if we believe God won't forgive us if we haven't forgiven others. It's almost amusing sometimes when people tell us they don't need to forgive anyone, but when we begin to minister to them, we find there are multitudes of people who have hurt them and need their forgiveness.

The truth is that every person on this planet, if they were to truly search their heart would find that they are in un-forgiveness because there are always people in our lives who have hurt or offended us and need our forgiveness. The problem is not with hidden unforgiveness, but how we deal with the known unforgiveness that brings the negative effects of guilt, shame and condemnation.

We must always remember that God came to redeem imperfect people, not to mention the fact that redemption couldn't even happen in your life without His forgiveness. God will never withhold His forgiveness, but your un-forgiveness may very well prevent you from receiving it. Unless you forgive from deep within your heart, you will live in guilt, shame and condemnation.

This in turn will prevent you from having faith in your heart to receive healing or answers to prayer. Forgiveness opens doors and un-forgiveness closes doors. It's our choice to open or close them between God and us, and between us and others. It's always our choice!

ALL OF US NEED FORGIVENESS FROM OTHERS AND OTHERS NEED FORGIVENESS FROM US

There is no such thing as a perfect person, parent, sibling, friend, boss, teacher or pastor. All of us need forgiveness from others, and others need forgiveness from us. We all have flaws, and all of us have had bad things done to us that we didn't need or desire. And all of us have had good things withheld from us that we did need. People have done bad things to us and we have done bad things to others. Therefore we all have people that are in need of our forgiveness, and we all need forgiveness from others for what we have done to them.

THE ONE WHO FORGIVES IS THE ONE WHO BENEFITS THE MOST

The offender may benefit from our forgiveness, but the one who forgives is the one who benefits the most, because we're set free from sin, guilt and condemnation. We're also set free from the torment of having the person who hurt us, along with the wrongs they did to us constantly replaying in our heads and hearts.

"When our hearts are free, we have confidence before God; and whatever we ask we receive from him, because we keep his commandments and do what pleases him." (1 John 3:21-22) NKJV.

It doesn't mean we have to be perfect in order to receive forgiveness from God. But it does mean that when our heart is free from guilt and condemnation and open to His desires, we are then in a far better position to receive what we need from Him.

Allow me to give you a word picture of our receiving all the things we need from God. Imagine if you will that you are outside in the rain, but because you are under an open umbrella you are staying dry and the rain is not affecting you. However if you were to lower the umbrella, you will get wet from the rain. It is much the same way with receiving healing or answers to our prayers. Receiving is a matter of posturing ourselves to receive, and part of that is to understand our God. God doesn't just save us, He is salvation! He doesn't just deliver us, He is deliverance! He doesn't just protect us, He is protection! He doesn't just heal us, He is healing!

Everything we need is found in Him. God is not God because of His actions, He is God because of Who He is. The Bible teaches us that He is not only in us, but He is also everywhere at the same time. This means everything we need for life is in us and is everywhere we may be, every moment of our lives. He is like the air we breathe which is in us and also everywhere we may be at all times.

Everything that we need is contained in His essence and is continually flowing from Him, just like rain falling from the sky. If we feel condemnation, shame or guilt due to unforgiveness or any other sin, it acts like an umbrella that prevents us from receiving what we need from Him. But when we confess our sin or in this case forgive others, it's like lowering the umbrella and all His goodness can flow unhindered to us, and we'll receive what we need.

Although, for many, especially the believer, a main umbrella is unforgiveness, there can be other umbrellas, such as unbelief, doubt, wrong teaching from pulpits, upbringing that has you believing you are unworthy, or believing He is an angry or uncaring God. We will cover some of these further on.

Often times the one we most need to forgive is ourselves. In the process of praying for people, many times we find that they are instantly healed after they have forgiven others or themselves.

We all have had wrong attitudes or

motives, and we all have made poor decisions or taken wrong actions. The problem is that we often believe we must pay for those sins, bad decisions or actions. It may be consciously or sub-consciously, but inwardly there is a feeling that we don't deserve to be healed. This often results in sending ourselves a message that our bodies must pay for our sins or poor decisions. This is all done on a sub-conscious level, but it still gives the devil an open door to bring sickness, because we have given him permission through our subconscious message that we must pay for our wrongs.

How many times have people been injured through a poor decision, such as trying to play tackle football or some other sport or action they should not have done. Their response is to say something like, "it's my own fault for being so stupid to try to do this,"

In doing so, they not only sent their bodies a message that was negative, but opened the door for the enemy to come in and produce some unwanted results, such as long lasting pain through their words. It may sound silly to talk to our bodies, but many times healing takes place when we have people apologize to their bodies for having sent it a subconscious message that their bodies had to pay for their sins, mistakes or bad decisions. We talk to inanimate objects like cars, street lights, or the person ahead of us at McDonalds because they are taking too long, none of whom can hear us. So why not talk to our living bodies and send them a new positive message. Why not tell our bodies that we like them and are grateful for all they have done for us, and give them permission to be healed and live a long, healthy, pain free life. Why not send our bodies a new message that they don't have to pay for our mistakes. It may sound silly, but we have found it works and many people are instantly healed as a result.

MANY STRUGGLE TO TRULY FORGIVE OTHERS OR THEMSELVES

People say, "I have forgiven so and so," but the fruit of true forgiveness is never evident, and they are still living in torment. Unfortunately wrong teaching has produced wrong results, and therefore many find it hard to authentically forgive others or themselves.

An overly simplistic idea has been promoted that forgiveness is merely an act of our will, therefore all we have to do is to forgive a person by an act of our will. Sounds great and easy, but that doesn't always produce true forgiveness, any more than someone speaking the "sinner's prayer" out of their heads and not out of their hearts will produce an authentic Believer. Our will is definitely involved, however all one has to do is look around and see that true forgiveness has never taken place. The offense never left, nor did negative and tormenting thoughts. Their heart is still wounded and full of pain.

Jesus gives us some insight of true forgiveness in the parable of the un-forgiving servant.

*"Shouldn't you have had mercy on your fellow servant just as I had on you? In anger his master handed him over to the jailers to be tortured, until he should pay back all he owed. This is how my heavenly Father will treat each of you unless you forgive your brother or sister **from your heart**.* (my emphasis) *(Matthew 18:33-35)* NIV.

There are several key truths that are found in this parable. Jesus is saying that until true forgiveness takes place, we'll be tormented or tortured in our minds and hearts. We have found in the process of ministering to countless people that the one who is tormented isn't the one who wounded them, but themselves. They are tormented in their hearts and minds as they continually remind themselves, like a broken record, of how the other person wronged them.

I recall many years ago how Ann Landers, a prominent columnist at the time, said these famous words, "why would you let your worst enemy live rent free in your head?" I have no idea if she was a Believer or not, but she was certainly in agreement with what Jesus taught. The one tormented is almost never the one who caused the wounding. Many times the one who caused the wounding isn't aware of how they hurt you or may not even care if they did hurt you. The tormented one is always the one who was wounded because they refuse to truly forgive.

The second major thought Jesus was trying to convey, is that true forgiveness in never just an act of our will, but must come from the heart. Please understand that God is not the one tormenting you. The consequence of your unforgiveness is the cause of your torment. Unforgiveness opens the door, and gives the enemy of your soul permission to torment you as he continually reminds you of the hurtful things the person did to you and how much suffering they caused you.

When Jesus said, that is how My heavenly Father will treat you, He isn't saying that God is causing the torment. However, God will never violate your free will! Jesus was saying that because we are free moral agents God must allow the consequences of our unforgiveness to take place in our life.

UNFORGIVENESS HAS CONSEQUENCES OF TORMENT

All sin, including unforgiveness has consequences. Jesus paid for our sin, but we have the responsibility to activate His work on the cross in our lives.

"If we claim to be without sin (sin of unforgiveness), **we deceive ourselves** *and the truth is not in us. If we confess our sins, He is faithful and just and will forgive us our sins and purify us from all unrighteousness."* (my insert and emphasis) *(1 John 1:8-9)* NKJV.

HOW DO WE FORGIVE FROM OUR HEART AND NOT JUST OUR HEAD?

So, the important question is, how do we forgive from the heart and not just from our head, so genuine forgiveness can take place and set us free from torment? In the parable of the unforgiving servant, Jesus gave us the answer to this question.

"The kingdom of heaven is like a king who wanted to settle accounts (recognize & realize fully what was owed) *with his servants. As he began the settlement, a man who owed him ten thousand bags of gold was brought to him."* (my insert) *(Matthew 18:23-25)* NKJV.

Although the king in the story does show the compassion of a forgiving God, he doesn't represent Father God. The king represents us, because Jesus is attempting to show that forgiveness can't come until we take a full account of what is owed us or done to us. True forgiveness can't come unless we fully comprehend and also acknowledge the whole scope of what someone has done to us, or in some cases what they withheld from us that we needed from them.

Many times people may forgive someone for what they did to them, but they never addressed how it made them feel or the long term affects it has had on their lives. A woman can forgive the act of her uncle sexually abusing her when she was a child. But forgiveness isn't complete unless she also forgives him for making her feel dirty, shameful and violated. The third ingredient is that she must forgive him for how it affected her life. An example is that she is fearful to get close to her husband, or as we often see the opposite happening, with some end up living in promiscuity. In ministering to wounded women we have seen both extremes in nearly all who have been sexually violated as a child. The great news is that they were all totally set free through authentic forgiveness. Genuine forgiveness does work!

FORGIVENESS MUST INCLUDE THE ACT, THE EMOTIONAL FEELINGS, AND THE LASTING EFFECTS ON ONE'S LIFE

To reiterate, because most people have been taught to only forgive the person, the forgiveness was never complete with the result the trauma and torment remained. True forgiveness must not only include the acts, but also the emotional feelings, as well as the lasting effects on one's life.

Another important ingredient is that the memory and trauma must be revisited in order to involve the heart and emotions for forgiveness to be genuine. This is necessary not only to forgive from the heart, but to also provide the opportunity for the Lord to bring healing to the pain and trauma involved. It's amazing how people have kept the pain and trauma stuffed and hidden from their conscious mind for many years. However, healing can only come when they're brought into the light. It can be very painful to revisit and reopen old wounds and trauma. However the good news is that the pain is only for a moment, while the effects of releasing that pain will last the rest of your life as you are finally set free.

We have found that much healing comes from the simple act of finally being able to vocalize to another person what has been stuffed and hidden for countless years. In the original Greek, the word for "confess" is the "homolegeõ" which is to acknowledge or agree with God about our actions, thoughts or motives. The Greek word for sin is "harmatia," which means to miss the mark or God's best. With this in mind, we can better understand what sin and confession is all about.

"If we say that we have not sinned (not missed the mark or God's best), *we deceive ourselves, and the truth is not in us. But, if we confess our sins* (agree with God and acknowledge that we have missed the mark or His best), *He is faithful and just to forgive us our sins and to cleanse us from*

all unrighteousness (to cleanse us from not doing what is right and good for our own benefit)." (my inserts). *(1 John 1:8-9)* NKJV.

"Is anyone among you sick? Let them call the elders of the church to pray over them and anoint them with oil in the name of the Lord. And the prayer offered in faith will make the sick person well, and the Lord will raise them up. If they have sinned, they will be forgiven. Therefore confess (acknowledge and agree with God) *your sins to each other and pray for each other so that you may be healed. The prayer of a righteous person is powerful and effective.* (my insert) *(James 5:14-16)* NIV.

Did you know that after the cross we are no longer required to ask for forgiveness? Forgiveness came for all our past, present and future sins when Jesus died on the cross. What we are to do is confess and repent. Without going into depth of the meaning in the Original language, the word "repent" is to revisit our actions and look at them from God's perspective of righteousness, agree with His assessment, and then do an about face and go in the proper direction. The word "confess" is similar and works in tandem with repentance in that it means to simply agree with God that our actions were wrong. After confession and repentance *"He forgives us and cleanses us from all unrighteousness."* Then the ball is back in our court. His forgiveness and cleansing must be **received!**

Forgiveness and cleansing is no longer something we ask for, but a matter of receiving. Like a mother holding out a cookie for her child. The child doesn't need to ask, but simply receive, and hopefully will thank his mom. It's like Christmas morning. You don't ask for presents, you simply open the gifts already under the tree and thank the person who gave them to you.

When Jesus died on the cross He gave us far more than we can ever imagine. We have so concentrated on using the cross to get to heaven, that we have overlooked all the many benefits He purchased for us to enjoy in this life while on earth. God won't throw rocks at you if you come crying asking for His forgiveness, any more than the mother would be upset if her child asked for the cookie already offered to him or her.

The wonderful truth is that God is already holding out the cookie of forgiveness to you and all you need to do is confess, repent and receive with thanksgiving and gratefulness. We don't have to beg for what He's already holding out to us. When we understand how really good God is, we'll automatically have a love affair with Him.

Can you see how hindrances such as wrong beliefs and unforgiveness can become large umbrellas and stop us from receiving all the things God wants to give us, besides all the things we need from Him?

Acknowledging the pain and trauma, forgiving and releasing the person from our judgment, along with giving the pain and trauma to the Lord, will set us free from the torment that has been in our life. Forgiving someone is never saying what the person did was right or okay. It also doesn't mean you must now be friends or have a relationship with them. What it means is that from your side, you have made peace with them and with God.

Unforgiveness in essence, takes God off the throne in our hearts, so we can play God by taking His place and becoming judge, jury and executioner over the one who hurt us.

UNFORGIVENESS IS TAKING GOD'S PLACE AND BECOMING JUDGE, JURY AND EXECUTIONER OVER THE ONE WHO HURT US

The truth is that only God has the authority, jurisdiction, knowledge, wisdom and power to judge properly, not to mention that He alone has the ability to see into the hearts and minds of people, and therefore able to properly execute justice or mercy.

"The word of God is alive and active. Sharper than any double-edged sword, it penetrates even to dividing soul and spirit, joints and marrow; it judges the thoughts and attitudes of the heart. Nothing in all creation is hidden from God's sight. Everything is uncovered and laid bare before the eyes of him to whom we must give account." (Hebrews 4:12-13) NIV.

Forgiving others is for your benefit so you can be set free from pain and torment.

However we often find that as people release their judgements against someone, God is set free to work in the offender's life to bring change for the good.

But, when we refuse to forgive a person there is a real sense in which we lock that person into the very thing that we despise about them and which prevents them from changing. When we forgive it opens up a potential for God to work in the person who hurt us, and bring change in their life for their good and our good.

FORGIVENESS SETS US FREE FROM TORMENT AND OPENS UP A POTENTIAL FOR GOD TO CHANGE THE ONE WHO HURT US

Recall the earlier thoughts on Quantum physics, where the particles of an atom would become what the physicist expected them to be. When we release our judgment to God and begin to have a better expectation for the person who hurt us, there is potential for change to come in them. Our freedom is the main goal, but the one who hurt us should also be important for two reasons.

First Jesus said we should love our enemies, which means we should want them to also find freedom.

Second, it could be doubly important if that person happens to be your spouse who you have to live with or your boss who you must interact with each day.

Nothing is ever restricted to us alone. We live among people and therefore we need to be at peace with everyone as much as possible. God's command to us is to speak and think well of and to people, even to the ones who hurt or offended us. That doesn't mean we can override their free will, nor does it mean we can practice witchcraft and control them. The key thought is that through your forgiveness, they will then have the "potential" to change. Through forgiveness and speaking well of and over them, the atoms that make up their being have the potential to change. Unforgiveness prevents potential and forgiveness allows potential to take place.

To sum it up, releasing judgment of others, along with forgiveness will set you free from torment and pain, and also have the potential to allow change to come to the one who hurt you. But, to reiterate, forgiveness is mainly for your benefit, not for the other person's benefit. You will be the one who is set free from torment.

A step we ask people to take when we minister to their wounded heart, is to have them picture the person in a prison cell. After asking Jesus for the key, we have them unlock the door and take the person by the hand and lead them out of prison. Then look them in the eye and tell them exactly how they wounded you, including how it made you feel and how it damaged and affected your life.

For example if you needed to forgive your dad, you would first say something like, "dad, thank you for bringing me into the world, for providing food, clothing and a roof over my head," but then go on to tell him exactly how he wounded you, along with the feelings and lasting affects his words or actions had on your life. "Dad, you wounded me deeply, when you............., but through the power of Jesus, I am forgiving you and releasing you from all of my judgment."

We don't recommend people physically go to the person, because their response may possibly be negative or cause more harm. They may not care if you forgive them or may argue with you over what they did. Our advice is to let God direct you.

The greater truth is that forgiveness is really between you and God. It is vertical action between you and God which has a horizontal impact between you and others. Forgiveness doesn't guarantee you will ever have a relationship with the person. But it does mean you will be able to live guilt free, and no longer be tormented in your mind and heart.

In revisiting the memories and going through the whole forgiveness process you also need to invite Jesus into the situation and the memories. As you experience the emotions and pain, this is the time to hand the pain, trauma and memories to Jesus, while picturing what He does with them in your imagination. Then ask Him to heal all the wounds and brokenness in your heart and mind.

The next step is to take the person and lead them to Father God, and say something like the following: "Father this person has hurt me terribly and to be truthful, I have wanted to see them punished for what they did to me. But, I have forgiven and released them from all my anger and resentment. I no longer want to punish them and no longer want You to punish them for me. What I am asking, is for You to set them in Your lap and put Your arms around them, and treat them like I wanted them to treat me. I am asking you to forgive and love them in the same way that I want You to forgive and love me. Amen."

I would like to leave you with another thought concerning forgiveness that Peter asked Jesus about.

"Lord, how many times shall I forgive my brother or sister who sins against me? Up to seven times? Jesus answered, I tell you, not seven times, but seventy-seven times." (Matthew 18:21-22) NIV.

The great news is that if God asks us to forgive someone 490 times a day, He would never ask us to do what He isn't willing to do for us. No matter how many times you or I sin, even 490 times a day, and confess 490 times a day He will forgive and cleanse us 490 times a day. That is really great news!

There is another aspect that is connected to forgiveness which needs to be addressed, and that concerns the effects that negative emotions have on health. The two major emotions that affect health are fear and anger which includes anxiety, hatred, rage, bitterness and resentment. In our physical bodies, we are neurological, chemical and electrical beings that operate in conjunction with our minds and emotions. Many major sicknesses are tied to either fear or anger. Heart attacks, asthma, thyroid, stomach problems, and others are often triggered by fear. Anger, including rage and hatred are the major contributors of some cancers, strokes, and many other major illnesses. Many of us have seen people turn red with rage, and we have thought or said, "he was so angry that his veins were bulging." In the healing ministry, it has been found that nearly all diseases have a spiritual root, with some kind of sin behind them, which is usually seen as some form of fear or anger.

Dr. Carolyn Leaf, a Christian brain scientist, has shown that anger, hatred and rage actually alters the brain in a very negative way. When we have emotions such as fear or especially anger, our neurological systems in conjunction with our electrical and chemical systems will be altered in a very negative way. When that happens chemicals and hormones are released that cause our immune system and other organs to shut down or not operate properly, resulting in sickness, disease and premature death. Sin will never stop God from loving us, but sin does have consequences, in the physical, spiritual and emotional realm.

Although all sicknesses and diseases have a spiritual or sin root we need to be very careful to not judge people. Just because someone has a stroke doesn't automatically mean they have a problem with anger or rage. A stroke can also be caused by weak artery walls, blockages, or other natural causes. There are also some sicknesses and diseases due to environmental conditions such as asbestos or radioactive material that can cause cancer and other problems. The caution is to never judge or condemn anyone.

In ministering to others, we always need to allow Holy Spirit to give discernment, but only for the sole purpose of seeing that person healed and set free, never for judgment, guilt or condemnation.

"Those who have not shown mercy will not receive mercy when they are judged. To show mercy is better than to judge." (James 2:13) NIRV

When praying for people to be healed, we should always expect God to move, but whether or not they instantly manifest their healing, the most important thing we can do for them is to leave them feeling guilt free, loved and extremely valuable to us and to God.

There is one last area we need to deal with and it is found in an amazing passage in Luke's gospel that addresses the impact on our lives as a result of our responses to how we have been offended or hurt by others.

"Judge not, and you shall not be judged. Condemn not, and you shall not be condemned. Forgive, and you will be forgiven. Give, and it will be given to you: good measure, pressed down, shaken together, and running over will be put into your bosom. For with the same measure that you use, it will be measured back to you." (Luke 6:37-38) NKJV

This is an amazing passage that has a far greater impact on our lives than we can imagine. Jesus truly meant what He said about what we give, we will receive back in greater measure, whether for good or bad. The Lord revealed that the truths found in this passage go much deeper than what first appears.

Wrong responses produce negative consequences that the enemy of our souls not only empowers, but most often keeps hidden to prevent us from finding freedom. At any moment in time someone is always getting hurt and wounded, which creates major harm or problems in their life. There is no way to deny it or sugarcoat the reality of pain and suffering that is inflicted and absorbed in a person's heart and life.

It isn't inclusive, but deep wounding usually occurs in a person's life when they are very young. It's an age when they're not able to defend against it or understand why it is happening. All they know is that they hurt and don't know why it's happening to them or what they have done to deserve such treatment.

As long as we're on this planet, we are prime targets with the potential to experience being wounded many times in our lives, no matter what our age may be, but it's more deadly when young. When we're young, we are most vulnerable. As we're developing, there are negative things that take place that have lasting consequences. All through life, parents, spouses, authority figures, and others, through their words and actions make negative judgements about us. Out of these judgments, they send us messages that we receive and begin to believe in our hearts. They can be varied messages such as stupid, unwanted, liar, untrustworthy or ugly.

These messages become labels that then

become our identities. We then begin to become and live out of those labels placed on us. Out of their judgments also come ungodly expectations placed upon us. In other words they expect us to be what they have placed on us. All this is in addition to the wounds they have inflicted upon us, which we must deal with. I hope you are beginning to see that we must sometimes go much deeper than simply making a choice to forgive a person.

To become free from what you just read, we must forgive them not just for the wounding, but, also for the judgments, messages, labels and ungodly expectations they have placed upon us. We must also come out of agreement with them and break their power off of us. This is not a book on healing of wounded hearts, but often it's connected and interwoven with physical healing. Therefore I felt it necessary to address enough so that the goal of physical healing is reached, which obviously is the main theme of this book.

I hope you can see that forgiveness is at times much more involved than what is proclaimed from too many pulpits. Too often guilt and condemnation is put on people by telling them, they should just forgive without any guidance. I hope you can see where the truths of the passage in Luke come into play in our lives, if we don't complete the process.

*"Judge not, and you shall not be judged. Condemn not, and you shall not be condemned. Forgive, and you will be forgiven. Give, and it will be given to you: good measure, **pressed down, shaken together, and running over will be put into your bosom.** For with the same measure that you use, it will be measured back to you."* (my emphasis) (Luke 6:37-38)

When we are hurt by anyone, there is a tendency for us to rise up in anger, hatred, bitterness or resentment, just to name a few. Hidden in the midst of these emotions are judgments, messages, labels and ungodly expectations that we then place on them for what they did to us. Please hear and receive this vital truth the Lord is revealing. Jesus said the judgments, messages, labels and ungodly expectations you have made against them, including your unforgiveness, will act like a boomerang and come back multiplied to you and go deep into your heart. The result is you will receive a life of judgment, labels and ungodly expectations placed deep into your own heart. It is a Biblical principle that we'll reap what we sow.

The answer is confession, repentance, and to break off what you have placed on them along with forgiving them. Remember that what's in our hearts is what determines what we will live by. I speak out of my own personal experiences, and have learned that when someone is judgmental or unforgiving towards me, the first thing I do is ask Holy Spirit to reveal if I have judged, used negative word curses, or placed labels, ungodly expectations, or have been un-forgiving towards anyone. I have learned that I will receive multiplied back what I have given. As it says in Galatians, we will reap what we sow, good or bad. To me it makes sense to sow a crop we want to eat.

In the appendix you will find a worksheet and specific prayers to help you deal with this area of forgiveness and judgments, along with other helps and prayers to bring freedom to have a full life that Jesus paid for on the cross.

THE TENSION, CONFUSION AND DISAGREEMENT OVER HEALING PRAYER

To anyone who has been in need of healing prayer, along with those who have had opportunities to pray for others, there seems to be a paradox or tension that leads to confusion, along with disagreement among Believers. And, it seems to be even more pronounced among those who would be labeled as "faith people." Obviously, all healing is received through faith, however when we speak of people in the faith camp, we're referring to those who believe that we have already been healed. And, that our healing will be evident or manifested as we believe and confess what has already been accomplished through Jesus Christ and His redemptive work on the cross. This belief is absolutely true and accurate as confirmed through many passages throughout the Bible in both the Old and New Testaments, and I totally agree with it. But, at issue is how it is handled in day to day life and application.

"Bless the LORD, O my soul, and forget not all His benefits: Who forgives all your iniquities and Who heals all your diseases." (my emphasis) *(Psalms 103:2-4)* NKJV.

It is important to note that the words "forgives" and "heals" are present and continuous tense verbs, meaning that God's forgiveness and healing is relevant for all times, including our present time. Some people believe and say that God exists outside of time, however that isn't totally accurate. It's more accurate to say the God is greater than time, and is present and active in all of time. We experience or view time much like looking through a knot hole in a fence at the parade of time going by, and are only able to see a small part at any given moment. But, from God's vantage point, it is as though He sits on top of the fence of time and is able to see the whole parade of time all at once. Not only is all of time present to Him, but, more important, He is present and active in all of time.

What the Psalmist was conveying is that no matter what time in history that you are alive, God's forgiveness and healing is available for us.

"Surely he has borne our infirmities and carried our diseases; yet we accounted him stricken, struck down by God, and afflicted. But he was wounded for our transgressions, crushed for our iniquities; upon him was the punishment that made us whole, and by his bruises we are healed." (Isaiah 53:4-5) NRSV.

Isaiah was prophesying what Jesus was going to accomplish through His redemptive work on the cross. The original language is clear in that it shows that Jesus was going to take our sins, infirmities, diseases, sickness and pains off of us, bear them on the cross and then take them to the grave to remain there forever. The deep truth is that if Jesus took our sickness and pains from us then we no longer have them.

This prophecy is repeated in the gospel of Matthew. It also must be noted that in both Isaiah's and Matthew's accounts, the words "bore" and "carried" are past tense verbs, meaning that in the eyes of God, Jesus has already carried or removed our infirmities, diseases, sickness and pains off of us, and bore them on the cross and left them in the grave.

"When evening came, many who were demon-possessed were brought to him, and he drove out the spirits with a word and healed all the sick. This was to fulfill what was spoken through the prophet Isaiah: "He took up our infirmities and bore our diseases." (my emphasis) *(Matthew 8:16-17)* NIV.

The apostle Peter further emphasizes that our healing has already been accomplished, and not something that is waiting to happen.

"He himself bore our sins in his body on the cross, so that we might die to sins and live for righteousness; by his wounds you have been healed." (my emphasis) *(1 Peter 2:24)* NIV.

What many believe is that the truth embedded in God's Word reveals that since our healing has already occurred, the manifestation of our healing will come as we believe in our hearts (not just our heads), and confess or declare that we have been healed. I totally agree with this truth, but it does cause some tension, confusion and disagreement among believers when it comes to receiving prayer for healing.

There seems to be a yes and no paradox or tension concerning healing prayer. There seems to be an unspoken question in some people about receiving healing prayer, even among those of us who consider ourselves "faith people."

According to the Bible we have already been healed, so the question or tension comes over whether we should have others pray for our healing or should we even pray for our own healing, or should we simply believe and thank God for having already healed us? The short answer is both yes and no! I will give you the no answer first.

The belief among many is that, in place of praying for God to heal us, instead we are to thank Him for having already healed us. Therefore as we believe and exercise our faith, manifestation of our healing will come, sometimes instantly, other times it may be hours, days or weeks. So, it follows that rather than having others pray for you to be healed, instead have them agree with you that you have already been healed, even if your symptoms of sickness or pain remain after the prayer of agreement. Many people would argue that we are lying if we are declaring we have been healed and the symptoms are still there. But Bible faith is declaring things that are not yet evident in the physical realm to be true and will come into being in the physical realm as verified by the Bible.

"God himself, who makes the dead live again and **speaks of future events with as much certainty as though they were already past."** (my emphasis) *(Romans 4:17)* TLB.

A great truth is that not only our healing, but every need we have, already exists in the invisible or in God's realm. Because God exists in all of time He knew our every need, including healing, and provided for them in the invisible or spiritual realm even before our world was created. In a very real sense, in God's world and in His eyes, the death of Jesus on the cross is in all of time, past, present and future. Which means all that He accomplished is in effect in all of time.

No man or woman since the fall meets the requirements of entrance into God's kingdom on their own merit or righteousness. When the redemption through Jesus was complete it covered all of time. Jesus and the cross of redemption happened and applied to all of time in the eyes of God. That's why the Old Testament saints looked forward to the cross. To God our needs are always present with Him before they ever exist or manifest in our physical realm. Like any good earthly father, our heavenly Father has already provided the answers that we need before we or our needs existed. The important point is that the answers we need are already created, and not something that has yet to be created or accomplished or something that we must convince God to do.

Not only does what we need exist, but in God's eyes we are already healed. The goal of faith and belief is to bring what already exists in the invisible or spiritual realm into our physical world. But, like many things of God, it must be contended for, before we can see them in our physical realm.

"We shall reap if we faint not or do not give up. So let us not grow weary in doing what is right, for we will reap at harvest time, if we do not give up." (Galatians 6:9) NRSV.

Jesus addressed His disciples about this when they saw how quickly the fig tree died after He cursed it.

*"If you only have faith in God—this is the absolute truth—you can say to this mountain 'Rise up and fall into the Mediterranean,' and your command will be obeyed. All that's required is that you really believe and have no doubt! Listen to me! You can pray for anything, and **if you believe,*** (heart belief) ***you have it; it's yours!"*** (my insert and emphasis) *(Mark 11:22;24)* TLB

William Branham was part of the major healing revival in the late 1940's through the early 1960's. His ministry was marked by many tremendous instances of miraculous healings. One such miracle concerned a man healed of blindness. Branham prayed for him, but the man responded by saying he was still blind. At which point Branham rebuked him and said, "do not say you are blind, but declare you can see." The man followed Branham's advice and began declaring to everyone he was around that "he could see," even as he was using his walking stick to guide him. His son was a barber and would cringe because his dad came into his barbershop every day and declared he could see. His son wanted to hide because everyone would laugh at his dad because all they could see was that his dad was still blind as a bat. However a few days later as he sat in his son's barbershop, his eyes suddenly popped open and he had perfect vision.

This a true story and was medically confirmed, illustrating how unwavering faith in the face of opposing evidence and opposing voices will produce in the physical realm what already exists in the invisible and spiritual realm.

Every authentic Bible scholar agrees that

God is all knowing. He never has a thought, nor has He ever had to come up with an idea. He simply knows all things at all times. That is hard for our human mind to comprehend, since our mode of operation, apart from direct revelation through Holy Spirit is to think before we can know something. But with God, knowing all things at all times is one of His natural attributes, just like His attribute of being omnipresent. Our challenge is we too often view God thru human lenses instead of through the eyes of Holy Spirit and His Word.

Authentic Bible faith is to believe the Word of God to be true even in the face of conflicting evidence. Bible faith is also not giving up until we receive what God has provided. The catch is that we must believe in our hearts, not just in our heads. I'm not saying that it's easy or without major challenges, but it's available for us.

The reality is that too often when people declare they have been healed, they aren't really believing but only hoping they will be or have been healed. Faith receives.

Hope, while vital, is not the same as true faith or believing that we have already received. Hope says it may be a possibility somewhere in the future, while faith declares we already have it. The key is that it must be heart belief and faith, not mere head knowledge that will bring forth the manifestation of healing. Too often people are only hoping that what they are speaking will come to pass.

There's no easy way to say this, but sometimes people sound like they believe and have faith to be healed, but that doesn't always mean they have authentic faith and belief in their heart.

"Above all else, guard your heart, for everything you do flows from it." (Proverbs 4:23) NIV

"Above all, be careful what you think because your thoughts control your life." (Proverbs 4:23) ERV

These two versions do an excellent job of giving us different slants at revealing what Solomon was attempting to convey. When he said to guard our hearts, he was saying that we need to be careful what we receive and allow to be placed in our hearts. The second version carries this further and reveals that what we put in our hearts will become our thoughts, our thoughts will become our beliefs and our beliefs will become our action, or in keeping with our subject, will determine if we live in faith or in doubt and unbelief, which will lead to failure.

Anyone can talk the talk and even put on a pretense of walking the walk, at least in public or when everything is going well. But the real test is what their talk and walk looks like when they face brick walls such as the giants of cancer, Aids or liver failure.

HOW CAN WE ACQUIRE BELIEF AND FAITH IN OUR HEARTS AND NOT JUST IN OUR HEADS?

I will attempt to answer an important question many believers have concerning faith and belief. The question is how can we acquire strong belief and faith in our hearts, and not just in our heads? First, please understand that I'm not coming from a platform of having come anywhere near to having arrived. I am far removed from having all the answers. Like many believers, there are times when I have struggles in the area of faith and belief. Some may never admit they struggle, but in truth, none of us have come close to walking in faith like Jesus did, in spite of all the WWJD bracelets we may wear. There are however, some practices that have made a huge difference for me, which I hope will also help you in your quest for greater faith and belief.

There may be some believers, like my wife who seem to be able to snuggle up to God in intimacy with very little effort. For me, it has always been a struggle and I have had to work at it. My challenge is that my mind appears to live in the midst of a ping pong tournament as the little plastic ball they are batting back and forth. Maybe some of you can relate. Something always seems to need my attention or things that I need to think about or find solutions for something. Needless to say, quieting my mind can be a battle in order to have a fighting chance for intimacy with God. Definitely a hindrance, but it has also caused me to be diligent and persistent in finding ways to quiet myself and find ways to connect with God and the Bible in intimate ways.

The good news is that God will always meet us where we are. God doesn't want clones, and on purpose created us with our own unique personalities. God is the One Who draws us to Himself so every one of us can have intimacy and be in genuine communion with Him, no matter our personality, who we may be or our present circumstances.

The normal answer from most pulpits is to "read the Bible, believe God and faith will come." Sounds too easy and too good to be true, doesn't it? It's a genuine truth, but also an incomplete answer.

"You say you have faith, for you believe that there is one God. Good for you! Even the demons believe this, and they tremble in terror." (James 2:19) NLT

There is a great deal of difference between believing in God's power and His other attributes, verses believing God is good and will use His power for you or your good. There is also a difference between believing He is good on your behalf and not just for others, especially if they appear to live more holy or righteous than you do. We can never go wrong by reading the Bible because it's God's word to us, and He can always speak to us as we read. However we must do more than simply read if we're discover the true God of the universe and build faith.

I am a faith person and totally agree with

their belief that we can absolutely believe and trust God's word to work in our life. But simply reading or even memorizing the Bible doesn't always automatically translate into faith, as can be seen in the lives of the Scribes and Pharisees. They were not only well read in what was written, but were also required to memorize the first five books of the Old Testament. However, the majority of them were full of pride and arrogance, faithless and enemies of Jesus. Sounds like some of the Pharisaical people we all know who pride themselves in their Bible knowledge and untested faith, doesn't it?

Those who say faith will come as we read the Bible are theologically correct, but not totally correct in how it's achieved. Faith can't come without reading the Bible, but there is more to the story that needs to be understood.

"faith comes by hearing, and hearing by the word of God." (Romans 10:17) NKJV

"faith comes from hearing the message, and the message is heard through the word about

Christ." (Romans 10:17) NIV

It helps to understand the original language in the above passages to grasp what Paul was attempting to communicate. There are two different Greek words that are translated as "word or words" in the Bible. The Greek word "Logos" is used to describe Jesus.

"In the beginning was the Word and the Word was with God and the Word was God." (Logos) (John 1:1) NKJV

The Greek word "logos" is always used to refer to either Jesus or to the Bible as God's written word to us. The other Greek word is "rhema," which is also translated as "word" in the New Testament. Although there are several Greek Lexicon definitions to be found, they don't always give a clear picture of what is meant. We can say we are reading God's word "logos," but that doesn't necessarily mean we are receiving God's "rhema," Receiving God's "rhema" is better understood to be receiving a revelation or heart knowledge of what God wants us to know about a truth in His "logos" word.

Have you ever been reading a passage in the Bible, and it felt like a new truth and understanding about what you were reading just leaped off the page? When that happened, you experienced revelation or "rhema." You may have read that passage hundreds of times, but in a Nano second, you suddenly had a deep understanding of a truth that you had never seen before. It became a truth deep into your heart. That is God giving you revelation knowledge.

Revelation or "rhema" is knowledge that is received in our hearts where it can build our faith, change our life, encourage us, or for use in ministering to others. Revelation never comes for head knowledge, but for heart changing knowledge.

AUTHENTIC FAITH ONLY COMES THROUGH REVELATION

In the Romans passage Paul was revealing that authentic faith only comes when we receive a revelation of a truth that comes through preaching or reading the Bible, or through Holy Spirit. Don't let the term revelation cause you a problem. Revelation is just a way to relate how God takes His truth and makes it heart knowledge instead of just head knowledge. Head knowledge puffs us up like the Pharisees, but heart knowledge will allow us to walk in faith and authority like Jesus.

When the Bible said that Jesus spoke with authority, the difference between His words and the words of the Pharisees was that they spoke out of their head knowledge, but Jesus spoke out of revelation heart knowledge, which came straight from His Father. That's the kind of knowledge I desire, how about you?

Reading the Bible is important and vital. However to bring us life, we must read to gain faith through revelation, not just to gain information or head knowledge. Sometimes we think revelation as being some kind of mystical experience, but revelation is simply coming into a greater understanding of God and His ways' and what we need to know in order to walk in His light and life. Another way of understanding the difference between "logos" and "rhema," is to say logos is about receiving information and knowledge, but rhema is more about receiving God's heart and message into your heart.

As an example, God desires us to receive a message and not just knowledge about the blind man being healed in the gospel of John 9:1-7. Logos reveals the facts of the miracle, but God desires us to receive "rhema" or a message from the story that will change us. Put yourself in the place of a man who had been born blind, never seeing a flower, trees, or faces of people. Imagine his emotions, and how life suddenly became a world of color and wonder, because he could now describe what he saw in ways that he couldn't have done before. But, a deeper message, and one God would like us to receive is that the blind man discovered a God Who was full of compassion and love for a man who was considered a sinner, worthless and a burden on society. God so valued this blind man that He sent Jesus to open his eyes and give him a new life. Do you think he would be a dedicated follower and lover of Jesus as a result of his encounter with the creator and God of the universe? God wants us to understand that same message is for us. A "rhema" word or revelation that He would like us to receive in that story is that God is telling us that it was His love and compassion for you and I, that sent Jesus to die on the cross to heal everything that is broken in us.

It would be very difficult to have faith to believe God would save, heal, protect or provide for us if we didn't believe He was compassionate, caring and loving. Like for the blind man, Jesus stopped at the cross to heal you! Seeking faith for healing, Romans

10 might be better understood to say, "faith comes by hearing and hearing by the "rhema" word or message of God, that He's a compassionate, caring and loving God."

With the concept that gaining faith must come through a revelation of God, His ways and His truths, it may be helpful to discover some things that hinder that objective, along with things that may help.

OUR LENSES AFFECT HOW WE SEE GOD AND INTERPRET HIS WORD

A hindrance that prevents us from receiving or believing that His Word will work on our behalf, can occur when our interpretation of the Bible is seen through distorted lenses. The lenses that we see life through are controlled by several factors, such as our family's belief system, how parents and other authority figures treated us in our childhood, along with traumatic events in our lives, especially in childhood.

Our lenses we developed in life affect how we see God and interpret the Bible. It's how we see God and interpret the Bible in our hearts, not just our heads that will determine our faith and belief. If we had abusive parents, we will view God and His word through those lenses. We may believe in our heads and say that God is good and loves us, but subconsciously, in our hearts it may be a different story. Subconsciously we may believe He will be abusive like our parents, or at the very least not protective or not really care about us. The result is that we'll have very little true or authentic faith to believe that He'll heal us or answer any of our prayers. Instead of faith, there is only a faint hope of a possibility that He will come through for us. Even then it's conditioned on whether or not He's having a good day and not ticked off at us.

When I was growing up, parents and other authority figures in my life were highly critical of me. When I became a believer, I felt God was just like them, and was always being critical of me. Of course like many believers, I said God loved and cared about me, but on a subconscious level was viewing God though my distorted lenses which crippled my faith and belief system. It wasn't until I received healing for the wounds in my heart, did I begin to interpret the Bible through lenses of a loving God, and discovered that He really is good and really loves and cares for me, and that He isn't angry or looking to catch me in some sin.

WRONG TEACHING DISTORTS OUR LENSES AND HOW WE SEE GOD AND HOW WE INTERPRET THE BIBLE

Next in degree of impact, is how wrong teaching distorts our lenses, and distorts how we see God and interpret the Bible. Not all preaching and teaching from Bible teachers, preachers or pastors is accurate or correct. Because we think of them as Bible authorities, we have a tendency to never question what they say. The result is we often receive everything as absolute truth, which is sometimes to our detriment. The reality is that a minister's teaching and preaching can sometimes be a product of their own faulty lenses which results in them having a distorted view of God and the Bible. Just because they are ministers, doesn't mean that they are immune to the same wounds others have suffered which can produce distorted lenses. When this is true in their lives, it can have a very detrimental effect on the messages they bring, and their effects on the listeners.

Another source of distorted lenses may have come to them through wrong or incorrect Bible training, which then perpetuated or introduce wrong beliefs in them and the messages they bring. I'm not saying we're to judge every minister or throw out everything they bring forth. What I am saying, is that it's our responsibility as the hearer to discern that what they're bringing forth is really Biblical truth. It's up to the listener to make sure the message and any passages they use are in agreement with the totality of what the Bible is saying, and that it also lines up with God's nature and His character. That includes everything I have written in this book. God gave us a brain and He would prefer that we use what He gave us instead of always relying on the voices or brains of others. We all need teaching, but we also need to make sure it's authentic truth and not a distortion of truth.

I attended a Bible college and seminary that belonged to a particular denomination, where they viewed God as being angry, judgmental, and that He constantly waited for us to sin so He could punish us or not answer our prayers. Their view of Christianity was based on a system that said, if you do the right things God is pleased and will help you, but if you do the wrong things, He will punish you and not be there for you or answer your prayers.

There is validity in the fact that there are always things we should do, along with things that we shouldn't do. But true Christianity is really about being and becoming, not about doing. Jesus did the doing so we could live as being and becoming.

When we discover and authentically live out of our true God given identity, righteous and holy actions will follow. We'll automatically live the authentic Christian life that God intends for us without effort. A mother duck doesn't have to teach her baby ducks how to quack, swim or waddle. Neither do baby ducks try to bark like dogs, crow like roosters or oink like pigs. They naturally and automatically quack, swim and waddle, because they automatically live out of their identity. True Christianity works the same way.

Some of this may seem foreign to you and off the subject, but rest assured, that until you begin to see through clean lenses, it will be difficult to see what God is really saying in His Word. Equally important is that with clean lenses, you will see the true God and not some distorted image of Him that has been painted through negative life experiences or wrong teaching.

Two major events took place when mankind fell in the garden. When man sinned, God never changed, but we lost the true image or identity of Who He is and began to see Him through sinful and distorted lenses, which brought a fear of God, among other things. We not only lost the true image of God, but equally important, we also lost our own Godly image or identity. A major work of the cross was to remove the sin factor for the purpose of restoring how we view God and His true identity. Equal to that was to restore our own true godly image or identity.

The good news is that God never stopped seeing us as His wonderful creations, so He sent Jesus to restore our ability to see ourselves the way He has always seen us. That is why we need "rhema" truth or revelation in our hearts to see ourselves as God sees us. When the truth of our identity enters our hearts, we'll see ourselves as God sees us. Then we will be like the baby duck and automatically become and live as authentic Christians.

We see this as Jesus attempted to bring this revelation to the Jews who had believed him.

"If you obey my teaching, you are really my disciples. Then you will know the truth. And the truth will set you free." (John 8:31-32) NIRV

From the passages prior to the above quoted verse and the ones that follow in John 8, show that the Jews in the above passage believed only part of what Jesus was saying. But they refused to believe that He was the son of God and their redeemer.

They had a distorted view of God and it stopped them from being truly set free.

No big secret, but there are many in churches today, including leaders, that not only have the wrong image of God, but are faithless because they are living out of a wrong identity, causing them to see through faulty lenses which prevent them from seeing and receiving truth.

Parents and others from our childhood, along with traumatic events in life, give us the lenses through which we view God and His Word. Therefore it's vital to make sure we are healed from the wounds in our hearts. As mentioned earlier, it may be necessary to also repent for wrongly judging God.

What follows are some practical steps that have helped me, and hopefully will help you build belief and faith in your heart. The first step is to stop reading the Bible as a task that needs to be accomplished. Reading the Bible is absolutely necessary in our lives, but I am against Bible reading plans as they are task oriented instead of God discovery oriented. I am a voracious Bible reader of both the Old and New Testament. However, I read to receive revelation and God's message for my life, and not just read to gain information or knowledge. I read with the idea of immersing myself in God and His message. When I was in Bible College and Seminary we were required to memorize many Bible passages, but that's no longer part of my life. To be honest, I have forgotten 99 percent of what they required us to memorize. The wonderful thing is that because I now read to discover Who God is and to find life in His Word, as I am ministering to someone or preaching, passages just flow out of my heart without effort or trying to memorize them.

The Pharisees memorized and were constantly in the Word, but the Word was never in them, and they never recognized the Living Word when He was among them. The Old Testament is good, but the New Testament is life. We are to learn from the Old Testament, but we are to live from the New Testament. I absolutely love the

Old Testament because it is so rich and has much to offer. I really love Psalms and often listen to an audio version while I sleep. However as good as it is and the help we can gain, it comes with a major caution. The high caution is that it's also about keeping rules and regulations. The Israelites were never able to keep the law and neither can we. Jesus came to fulfill the law and usher in the New Testament, which is all about grace and living out of a new identity, which results in freedom and authentic Christianity.

IMMERSE YOURSELF IN THE BIBLE TO BRING FAITH

One way you can immerse yourself into the Bible is by picturing yourself in the scenes and circumstances as Jesus ministered and dealt with life. As an example, put yourself in the cripple's place at the pool of Bethesda. What would you be thinking as you felt strength flow into your legs when Jesus told you to rise up and walk? How would you feel about your self-image because you could now work and live a normal life without begging for a living? How would you feel if you were no longer considered a sinner and a drag on your family? What would your emotions be if Jesus came back to you and said to stop your sinning so things will not go worse with you? Would you be offended, angry or repentant?

For the correct answer to how you would react to Jesus, is found in how you react in your present life. How do you react when someone in your life corrects you in front of others, points out your flaws or wrong actions (sins)? This answer may really be your true reaction if you were the cripple. I know. Ouch!

How would you feel if you were the prostitute after Jesus saved you from being stoned? How do you feel when you commit a major sin in your present life, and then Jesus pours His love and forgiveness into you? As you read, ask Jesus questions. Jesus, what were You feeling when Your own brothers and sisters didn't believe in You and thought You were crazy? Jesus, how does it make You feel when I don't believe what You say in Your Word is true for me or when I don't believe You will answer my prayers or don't believe You were there when I needed You? I know, ouch again! I have listed a few possible ouches, but that is only to bring some reality to what I am suggesting.

The Bible is full of comfort and love for you to discover. Do you get the drift? The goal is to immerse yourself in the Bible to build a relationship with the Godhead through

His Word. Reading the Bible as a task to accomplish will leave you dry and empty. When we read to discover the true God, and not the God that religion or religious teaching has manufactured, we will begin to truly know our wonderful God. We will begin to build genuine faith to move mountains.

PRAYING THE WORD
WILL REVEAL TRUTH IN
THE WORD TO YOU

Praying the Bible is another method I use. Not that it's wrong, but I don't mean to just pray the written words. Personalize it and thankfully pray it back to God. As you do, God and His truth will come alive in your heart. Praying the word will also bring revelation of truths that God wants to be instilled in your heart. I will list some verses and then show how I may repackage them as prayers to pray back to God. I have also recorded some of these repackaged prayers of Bible passages which address truths that can help me in life. I then play them at night while I sleep and find that the truths become a part of me without effort. Remember we highly value our own voice more than the voices of others. I want to repeat again, please stop reading the Bible as a text book and begin to live in it, not as an outsider, but as an insider and participant.

When I read, I also attempt to read everything in the first person. As an example, instead of reading Ephesians 1:11 as saying *"in Him we have obtained an inheritance,"* I will read it to say "Thank You Jesus for giving me an inheritance in You."

Misty Edwards wrote a song some years ago that said, *"I don't want to talk about You as though You are not in the room. I want to look right at You, and sing right to You."* The goal of Bible reading should be face to face communion with God! You can also take that passage as a prayer and say, "Thank You Father, for providing a way for me to obtain an inheritance in You through Jesus." This method helps to make the Bible become living truths to you and not just endless reading without purpose. If you have singing ability it would be a great method to use as you sing your repackaged prayer passages over yourself and back to God. God's word is alive, but it's our responsibility to do our part to have it come alive to us and in us.

The following passage is a favorite of mine, because it says that our true identity has been restored. It is important to understand that we're no longer sinners and enemies of God.

"Once you were alienated from God and were enemies in your minds because of your evil behavior. But now he has reconciled you by Christ's physical body through death to present you **holy** *in his sight,* **without blemish and free from accusation**--*as you continue in your faith, established and firm, and do not move from the hope held out in the gospel."* (my emphasis) *(Colossians 1:21-23)* NIV.

I might personalize this passage into a prayer by praying something like: "Father, I am so thankful to You for rescuing me from my old life. It's true that I was once Your enemy in my way of thinking and in my actions, but I'm so grateful to You for sending Jesus to die for me, so that You now see me as holy and without blemish, and free from all accusations or condemnation."

As you turn the Bible into personalized prayers of thanksgiving back to God, the truth He wants you to have will enter your heart, and you will be set free as Jesus spoke in John 8.

There was a man on television many years ago who could quote the entire New Testament and most of the Old Testament. The sad aspect was that like the Pharisees of old, he wasn't a believer. He knew the words of the Bible, but didn't know the God of the word. The apostle Paul said that, *"the letter kills, but the Spirit gives life." (2 Corinthians 3:6)* NIV

Authentic confession must come from authentic belief and faith which lives in our hearts, in order to be to be saved, healed or delivered. I recommend many of the passages in Romans 5, 6 and 8, Galatians, Ephesians and Colossians as scripture for personalizing into prayer. They are important passages that speak about God's identity, our identity, and who and what we have in God through the work of His Son Jesus on the cross.

Even what some would call negative

passages can be turned into prayers of thanksgiving. In Ephesians 4, Paul tells us *"do not be angry, do not sin, and not to use foul language."* You can turn it into a positive prayer by saying, "thank You Father, that I no longer live in anger, steal or use foul language because Jesus has set me free from my sin nature."

Although what follows is a list of passages on healing, my conviction is that they are secondary to discovering and living out of your God given identity. I truly believe our identity or more precisely, what we believe about our identity is the driver of our lives. What we believe about our identity will result in a life that can be either good or bad, because we will become and live out of who we think we are. It is important to immerse ourselves in what God has to say about healing. But, if we don't live out of our true Godly identity we'll not be in a position to receive healing because of guilt, condemnation, or feeling unworthy of receiving anything from God.

Some say that it doesn't matter who others say who you are, but only who God say you are. That is only a partial truth, because it's not even who God says you are. It's not until you **believe** and **accept** what God says about you that really matters. It's who you think or believe you are that will determine the quality of your life.

Following are some healing passages. However, once you discover the goodness of God, you will discover that healing is throughout the Bible and will find multitudes of passages that support God's desire to heal everyone. (Psalms 103:1-5, Psalms 103:20, Isaiah 53:4-5, James 5:14-16, Matthew 8:17, Mark 16:17-19,20, 1 Peter 2:24).

Please understand that it's not any particular style of prayer that matters as you pray the Bible back to God. It's a matter of the heart, so it's important to use words and a style of prayer that you are comfortable with. Simply talk to God as a friend, as an insider and not as an outsider. The purpose is never to impress God, get His attention, or even get Him to do something for you. The wonderful truth is that you already have His attention and

He's already impressed with you. And He has already done everything He needed to do for you through the work of Jesus on the cross.

A personalized prayer process is for you. As truth enters your heart you'll not only finally realize your true identity, but it will also help you to acquire true heart belief and faith instead of just head knowledge.

SOAKING BRINGS INTIMACY, REVELATION AND FAITH

Although I highly recommend and am a student of meditating on the Bible, would like to suggest another method for achieving intimacy with the Lord. Soaking can be a very useful method and helpful practice that can be integrated with immersing yourself in the Bible and praying God's Word back to Him. Soaking can bring intimacy, faith and revelation. If you aren't familiar with the term, it's best described as becoming quiet and putting yourself in a position of rest before the Lord. It's not a time for praying, petitioning or interceding. Praising and worshipping God may come into play, however the main objective is to quiet ourselves before God so He has an opportunity to invade our personal life without any preconditions or agendas.

It's a time of devoting yourself totally to Him in the quiet place of your heart. This is difficult for me because I have such a busy mind, but have found it can be done. It takes a willful decision to not only set aside a time every day, but to continually quiet your mind as it wanders, because wander it will. When it wanders, simply bring it back to God, whether through a few words of worship or quietly and reverently speaking His name.

God won't condemn you for losing focus, but will reward you for your efforts to refocus. Also, don't be concerned if you drift off in sleep, as God can and will speak to you while you sleep. Some people do well soaking in absolute silence. I find that soft instrumental worship music without words seems to work best for me. Music with words can sometimes be a distraction because of the temptation to sing along with the music. The purpose isn't to have a time of praise and worship, but to quiet ourselves before our God without distraction. Worship isn't for God, but for us. God is totally complete and needs nothing, including worship. Worship is really an opportunity to intimately connect with Him.

Giving Him our undivided attention is probably the greatest worship we can offer. Our goal is to give God an opportunity to invade our busy world. We want to shut the world out to meet with our Lord. There is no set time requirement. Some may spend an hour, while others may lie still for four or more hours.

Like Bible reading, soaking before Him should never be turned into a task or duty to perform. It's just another way to open our hearts to meet with our Father God without distraction. It's a way to say to God, "I don't want anything from You, I just want to spend time with You." Women, how would you feel if your husband came to you and said, I don't want anything, I just want to spend time with you? Even being a man, if my wife said that to me, my heart would melt. We are made in His image and likeness. He may be the creator and God of the universe, but He has the same emotions as we do. Give it a try. You may just melt God's heart. The Toronto revival in the 1990's was attributed to how

John and Carol Arnott, the leaders, would spend four hours every morning soaking before the Lord. The result was a revival that impacted the world, not just Canada.

Integrating soaking, Bible meditation and immersion, along with praying His Word back to Him has a great potential to bring change, faith, revelation, our true identity in God, and direction for life.

HEALING OFTEN COMES IN THE FACE OF CONFLICTING EVIDENCE

Many years ago, in the early 80's a man came to a meeting in severe pain because of kidney stones. A few years previously he had been operated on for the same problem, but they had returned along with tremendous pain. He had gone to the doctor and they scheduled him for an operation within a few days. The man didn't want to go through the painful operation again, and had faith that he would be healed if we prayed for him. We prayed, but nothing changed in the natural. But, in his heart he believed God's Word was true, and that he was healed even though he was still in excruciating pain. Through the years, we have learned that healing often comes in the face of conflicting evidence.

When he went to the hospital the next

day, he told the doctor he wouldn't allow them to operate until another x-ray was taken. He told the doctor he believed God healed him and that He wouldn't need the operation. The doctor at first refused, because they had just taken an x-ray three days prior, which showed the kidney stones along with scar tissue from the previous operation. In those days, they cut the kidneys open to remove the stones, which wasn't a pleasant ordeal. The man stood his ground and refused to have the operation without a new x-ray. The doctor reluctantly had a new x-ray taken, mainly to prove him wrong, and so they could begin the operation.

All the while this was going on the man was doubled over in pain, yet he refused to doubt God's Word. He firmly believed he was healed as a result of our prayers in spite of the pain. The doctor stuck the original x-ray on the viewing glass and smirked as he showed the man the scar tissue and kidney stones. But, when he placed the new x-ray on the glass, the doctor's mouth fell open because there was no sign of kidney stones or the scar tissue from the previous operation. Only at that instant did the man's pain leave!

Don't overlook this truth. If the man had doubted the Word of God he would have lost his healing. He was healed the instant we had prayed, but the devil did his best with lying symptoms to convince the man that he wasn't healed. Instead of being moved by or believing the lying symptoms he chose to believe and trust God's word. Like the blind man who was healed under William Branham's ministry, it was necessary for them to proclaim the truth of their healing in the face of lying symptoms.

God often works through others to bring healing, but you can receive your healing directly from God. Receiving it directly from God is actually the best way to be healed. It's better because you won't lose your healing because it's a result of your own strong belief and not dependent on another's faith.

Our faith is the opportunity to receive the promises of God in our lives. You may disagree with this statement but, **"The Word of God in your mouth has the potential to have as much power as the Word of God in God's mouth!"**

We are God's representatives on earth and charged with bringing His kingdom to earth as Jesus taught us in the Lord's prayer. He commanded us to lay hands on the sick, and when we do He will confirm our actions with signs (miracles and healing). (Mark 16:15:20).

Your prayers will bring results for you and others if you will only believe it and act in faith. I challenge you to stop reading and lay the book down, and lay hands on yourself if you need healing. Rebuke and command whatever sickness, disease or pain to leave in the name of Jesus, and command whatever is wrong to be healed in the name of Jesus Christ of Nazareth.

"Banish fear and doubt! Remember that the Lord your God is with you wherever you go."(or whatever you do) (my insert). *(Joshua 1:9)* TLB

RECEIVING PRAYER AND MANIFESTING YOUR HEALING CAN BRING TENSION

Receiving prayer and manifesting your healing can bring tension, because two different aspects are involved. And, this is the area where many people miss their healing.

"Is anyone among you sick? Let them call the elders of the church to pray over them and anoint them with oil in the name of the Lord. And the prayer offered in faith will make the sick person well; the Lord will raise them up. If they have sinned, they will be forgiven. Therefore confess your sins to each other and pray for each other so that you may be healed. The prayer of a righteous person is powerful and effective." (James 5:14-16) NIV

A great truth is that when someone prays for you to be healed, it's impossible for nothing to happen! Something always happens! The tension comes when the pain or condition doesn't immediately change. To be honest, many in the healing ministry including myself have unintentionally helped perpetuate the belief that healing didn't take place if nothing instantly changes.

The prayer model often used after prayer is that the person is asked to do something they couldn't do before prayer, such as bend over or move an immobile arm or leg, or to see if the pain level was diminished. It's a Biblical model. In the individual recorded healings, Jesus asked them to do what they could not do. Jesus asked the crippled man at the pool of Bethesda to take up his bed and walk. He asked the cripple who was let down through the roof to rise up and walk. He asked the man with the withered arm to stretch forth his hand. I want to say that with most of the people we pray for something always happens such as pain is eliminated or diminished, broken backs healed or deaf ears opened. The challenge comes when nothing changes, and people will sometimes walk away believing that they weren't healed.

Bethel has a major healing ministry where people come from all over the world to be healed. I have witnessed some absolutely amazing instant miracles such as cancers disappearing, blind eyes opened, deaf ears opened, and metal dissolving in backs, just to mention a few. But, it's also true that there were many people who were totally healed but didn't manifest their healing immediately. For some, their healing came hours, days, weeks and even months later. But the good news is that they were healed!

In the passage in James, the original Greek words that are used allude to healing that wasn't always instant. Even with Jesus, there were times, such as with the ten lepers who weren't healed instantly, but were healed as they walked, which was nearly a day's journey according to some Bible scholars. In another story of progressive healing, Jesus said to the nobleman,

"Go your way; your son lives." "So the man believed the word that Jesus spoke to him, and he went his way. And as he was now going down, his servants met him and told*

*him, saying, "Your son lives!" Then he inquired of them the hour when he **began to get better**. And they said to him, "Yesterday at the seventh hour the fever left him." So the father knew that it was at the same hour in which Jesus said to him, "Your son lives."* (my emphasis) *(John 4:49-53)* NKJV.

When the nobleman was told by Jesus to go his way for his son was healed, he learned through his servant, that his son **started to get well** yesterday, the day the centurion met Jesus, which was at least a day's journey.

If you're the one praying for someone, they always need to be assured that healing always comes forth from God in answer to prayer. And if you're the one being prayed for, be assured your healing did come forth from God. It may not be manifested in the natural as yet, but in God's invisible realm, it has already occurred.

One thing we emphasize is that even if the condition only improved 5%, we always encourage the person to be thankful for the 5%, and not even pay attention to the

95% that didn't yet manifest. We have found that, as they thank God for what they did receive, they are making the way for the full 100% healing to manifest. In being thankful for even partial healing, you are acknowledging and agreeing with God's Word, which says that you have already been healed.

Agreeing with the word of God is the very essence of faith. Faith is believing what God says to be true in the face of opposing evidence.

"Faith is the substance of things hoped for, the evidence of things not seen." (Hebrews 11:1) NKJV

Faith is not only a substance that brings things from the invisible realm into our physical realm, but is the evidence which validates that we believe what we need already exists in the invisible realm. It's like being physically blind, and someone tells you to sit down because there is a chair behind you. Because, you have faith in the person's words you choose to sit down. But you will never experience the reality or manifestation of the chair until you attempt to sit.

Faith isn't mystical. Faith is believing that God and His word are true for you no matter what it appears to be in the natural realm, and then your faith is validated by taking appropriate actions of trying to do what you couldn't do before.

We always want instant manifestations, but in the long scheme of things, who cares if it takes hours, days or weeks? People spend thousands of dollars and weeks, months and even years going to doctors without giving up faith in their doctor. A doctor gives someone a prescription to cure a problem, but the person doesn't say the doctor's word doesn't work before they even begin taking the medicine. Should we give up faith in God's Word so quickly before His Gospel (God's prescription) has a chance to work? People trust doctors despite the fact that the success rate of the medical profession is ridiculously poor, and would scare people away if they knew how bad it was. Shouldn't we give ourselves a little time to receive a full manifestation when we go to God?

The awesome truth is that nothing God ever spoke has failed. Our healing has already occurred in God's invisible realm over two thousand years ago.

At times there may be open doors that allow the enemy to delay or completely stop the manifestation of healing. The demonic realm will try to get involved through doubt, wrong teaching or wounding from childhood, which often gives us a wrong view of God and ourselves. And satan will do his best to ride shotgun alongside previously mentioned hindrances like unforgiveness, sins, curses, iniquity in our bloodlines, witchcraft, not to mention environmental and food issues.

Have you ever wondered why a person can live right, eat right and be sick, yet an unbeliever lives, acts and eats terribly but lives to a ripe old age full of health? It's because the enemy already knows he owns them and they are walking dead on their way to hell. Therefore he places his attention on us as he tries to kill, steal and destroy God's kids, so they are miserable on earth.

The point that's being made is that if healing seems to be delayed, we need to go to Holy Spirit who searches and knows all things to see if it's something in us such as unforgiveness or some other sin that may be bringing guilt and condemnation, or search to see if we need to deal with the demonic realm.

We deal with the demonic realm by directly taking authority over them, and by closing any doors that have given them permission to delay or stop the healing from manifesting. God always answers our prayers instantly, but sometimes it may take us time to understand what is stopping our answer so we can take the next step. If something isn't working, we need to ask Holy Spirit for His wisdom until He shows us what to do to change the situation.

"If you don't know what you're doing, pray to the Father. He loves to help. You'll get his help, and He won't be condescending to you when

you ask for it." (James 1:5) MSG

If the healing never comes we can be sure of two truths. First, we can be sure it's never on God's end. God sent His son to die for our complete healing in our spirits, souls and bodies. He already sent His word to heal and His word never comes back void, meaning His power and authority is attached to His word and cannot be separated from it. The issue is always on our end. It is either in us, the devil attacking us because he hates us, or a combination of us and him that is stopping the manifestation of our healing.

If we're healed, but if the pain or other symptoms come back, it isn't because God didn't heal you. The devil will come with lying symptoms to see if you will take his bait, so you will start thinking or saying, "I must not have been healed" or "I have lost my healing." When you do that you have just opened the door for the devil to give you the genuine deal back. Your response should always be *"By His stripes, I was healed."(1 Peter 2:24)* Fight back and command the devil and the pain to leave!

Unfortunately most of the church believes in a big devil and a small God, and then wonders why they live defeated lives. Satan is no match for God. He's like an ant under the wheels of a giant locomotive. When God spoke about the war in heaven when satan and his angels were kicked out, it happened in a Nano second with no effort on God's part. And the same thing will happen when Jesus comes back to battle satan and his army. God never was and never will be worried, intimidated, alarmed or concerned about satan. God is supreme over satan and He's supreme over your disease, sickness or pain.

"God lifted him up to the highest place. He gave him the name that is above every name" (Philippians 2:9) NIRV

The name of Jesus is above every name, and that includes the names of cancer, diabetes, ALS, MS, Alzheimer's, blindness, deafness, heart attacks, dementia, AIDS, and all names of sickness and disease. Every name must and will bow before His name that is above every name. We carry the power and authority of Jesus

Christ and when we pray in faith according to His Word, the mountains must move. God's Word guarantees that He will answer every prayer that's based on a promise in His Word. The promise of healing was signed, sealed and delivered by the death of Jesus on the cross. When Jesus said *"it is finished."(John 19:30)* they were not pitiful last words of relief that His suffering was over. In the original Greek the word Jesus spoke "it is finished," is the word "teleo."

It was a military word or term that would be used in the midst of a battle. In Bible days, battles were fought in hand to hand combat. Thousands of soldiers on a field fighting hand to hand, with their mind on the one objective, kill the man in front of them or be killed. If they were to take their eyes off their enemy for an instant, they would face death from an enemy who was looking for an opening to strike. They had absolutely no idea whose side was winning the battle. But! The commanders of each army would attempt to position themselves on high ground so they could effectively direct their troops. From this position they could determine who was winning. If a commander saw his side was winning, he would yell out ("teleo") it is finished! We have won the war! His troops would hear and surge forth with renewed strength, while the enemy would begin to flee in defeat. When Jesus cried out "It is finished," it was a war cry of victory and the enemy of our souls knew he was defeated.

The war has been won! The centurion standing by the cross was familiar with military language and understood exactly what Jesus meant.

*"Jesus cried out with a loud voice, and gave up His spirit. **When the centurion, who stood by opposite him, saw that he cried out like this** and breathed his last, he said, "Truly this man was the Son of God!"*(my emphasis) *(Mark 15:37,39)* WEB

In that epic moment the promise of healing was endorsed and ratified in His blood of the New Covenant, and declared to forever be in force and available for every man, woman and child. God's work of redemption for your spirit, soul and body is finished and available to you. There's nothing more God can or needs to do. What you need is waiting for you to appropriate in faith just like you did for your salvation.

RECEIVING PRAYER
MORE THAN ONCE ISN'T
A LACK OF FAITH

Now for the yes answer to receiving prayer, and whether you should have others pray for you more than once. As mentioned earlier, there are many ways to receive your healing, and although simply believing you are healed is the best way, it may not be the best way for you at the present time. Your answer may be for God to heal you another way. There is never a time or place for you to feel guilty or less than spiritual in your quest for healing. Receiving prayer more than once is not a lack of faith. It is demeaning and unloving to tell anyone they don't have enough faith to be healed.

"Because of his kindness, you have been saved through trusting Christ. And even trusting is not of yourselves; it too is a gift from God." (Ephesians 2:8) TLB.

The truth is that we all have a measure of,

and sufficient faith to be healed.

"For I say, through the grace given to me, to everyone who is among you, not to think of himself more highly than he ought to think, but to think soberly, as God has dealt to each one a measure of faith." (Romans 12:3) NKJV.

I like Peter, because he says everyone has the same amount and quality of faith that he had. Think about that. Peter is the one who preached on the day of Pentecost and 3000 were saved. People were healed when they came within a shadow length of him. (No, it was not his shadow as many preachers say. It was a Hebrew idiom meaning a shadow length. In our language we would say that when the people came close (a shadow length) to the anointing that he carried they were healed. There were also other accounts of Peter healing people in the book of Acts. The point is that we have the same faith he had.

*"Simon Peter, a bondservant and apostle of Jesus Christ, To those who have obtained **like precious faith** with us by the righteousness of our God and Savior Jesus Christ." (my*

emphasis) *(2 Peter 1:1)* NKJV

In the Original Greek, the word "like" is "isos," and it means equal in quality and equal in quantity. Surprise! You have enough faith!

Where the challenge for many is in the area of belief. Jesus said all we need is a mustard seed size faith. The truth is we have far greater than mustard size faith. If we can begin to truly believe what God and His word says, we will begin to operate in the mountain moving faith we already possess. It's a matter of belief!

If a stranger walked up to you and said, "if you will kindly walk to the bank with me, I will give you one million dollars in new one hundred dollar bills with no strings attached." You would be thinking, "yeah right, and I will sell you the Empire State Building for two dollars." Or some other thought that indicates you didn't believe him or think it couldn't possibly be legitimate. It isn't a matter of faith, but of belief. If you believed the man was truthful and you could trust him, you would exercise your faith and follow him to the bank.

When His disciples asked Jesus why they couldn't cast the demon out of the boy, He told them it was because of their unbelief. These same disciples had just come back from the places Jesus had sent them, where they were casting out devils and healing the sick. They were full of faith! It was a matter of unbelief. Jesus answered their question by saying that the only way they could get rid of their unbelief was through prayer and fasting.

"However, this kind does not go out except by prayer and fasting." (Matthew 17:21) NKJV

We have enough faith to move mountains, because we operate with the faith of God which is a gift to us. Even Jesus could only heal a few sick people in His own home town?

*"He could do no mighty work there, except that He laid His hands on a few sick people and healed them. And He marveled because of their **unbelief**. Then He went about the villages in a circuit, teaching."* (my emphasis)

(Mark 6:5-6) NKJV.

In this passage, Jesus was simply stating a fact, and not condemning them over their lack of faith. Instead of condemnation, he went about teaching them in order to strengthen their "belief," so they could be healed. He didn't say they had no faith, but had unbelief.

Authentic Biblical teaching and preaching is meant to build people up, not condemn them or tell them what is wrong with them. There is nothing wrong with going for prayer more than once. Jesus prayed for a blind man more than once. In the story of the man with an epileptic son, the disciples of Jesus couldn't cast the demon out, so the man came to Jesus for help. Jesus didn't rebuke the man or tell him he couldn't receive more prayer because the disciples already prayed for him. He simply asked him to believe and the boy was healed. The man not only sought additional prayer, but even admitted he needed help to believe. Jesus met him where he was at in his faith and belief without condemnation. If you feel you need to be prayed for a hundred times, do it without feeling guilty, condemned or lacking faith.

A Critical guideline! The critical guideline for receiving prayer more than once, is that each time you go for prayer, you must go with the belief that, "**This time**, I believe I will be healed when they pray, even if symptoms remain!" Not hope so or maybe. Just hoping you will be healed is like hoping you will win the lottery jackpot without buying a ticket. It won't happen! My encouragement is that in between going for prayer is to immerse yourself in Bible passages that address your identity in Christ, and in the multitudes of healing passages to build up your faith.

Please don't feel condemned, guilty or that something is wrong with you. We're all in process. No one has arrived. It's just that some are able to put on a better show than others. Here is what I encourage you to do as you build your faith. Use every avenue available to receive your healing. For you it may mean you will be healed by being in an atmosphere of healing where the presence of God shows up and people are healed even without prayer. It may mean you will be healed by someone operating in the gifts of faith, healing, miracles or words of knowledge. The point is that I encourage you to pursue your healing with determination and not give up until your healing is manifested.

God sent Jesus to procure your healing. Like money in your personal bank account, healing is available for you to draw it out of heaven's bank. It's your healing to receive by any and every means that will work best for you.

DEALING WITH HIDDEN BLOCKAGES

When you know there's something that's stopping you from receiving your healing, but you can't seem to put your finger on it, it may be an indication that you may need help, and have to look beyond yourself. There are times when we reap the results of previous generations because of their sins and iniquities that have been passed down.

"As he went along, he saw a man blind from birth. His disciples asked him, "Rabbi, who sinned, this man or his parents, that he was born blind?" "Neither this man nor his parents sinned," said Jesus, "but this happened so that the works of God might be displayed in him. (John 9:1) NIV

What is often missed, is the fact that the disciples well understood that the sins from previous generations are sometimes the cause of our physical problems. Jesus was simply pointing out that it wasn't the source of this particular man's blindness, yet at the same time didn't discount that this can be the case at other times. The actions of previous generations can have negative or positive effects on future generations.

"You shall not bow down to them nor serve them. For I, the LORD your God, am a jealous God, visiting the iniquity of the fathers upon the children to the third and fourth generations of those who hate Me, but showing mercy to thousands, to those who love Me and keep My commandments. (Exodus 20:5) NKJV

We have ministered to countless people who have had ancestors who were satanists, warlocks, witches, Freemasons, or involved in the occult in some way or fashion. We have found that Freemasonry in particular, (though often viewed as an innocent group), is often responsible for many unexplainable diseases and sicknesses. What many outsiders and those in the lower ranks of Freemasonry are ignorant of is that they are pledging allegiance to satan. It's not until they reach the higher ranks do they understand that they're worshipping satan, but then they are hooked because of the vows they have taken.

"Like a fluttering sparrow or a darting swallow, an undeserved curse does not come to rest. (Proverbs 26:2)

What isn't stated in this passage, but implied, is that a curse that is deserved can come and have an effect on us. This means not only our actions, but also our ancestor's sins or iniquities can give a curse permission to come upon us. In our Western world it isn't obvious, but in many countries people understand the power of curses. In our Western world and mindset, we often are oblivious to them, but still see the effects through diseases and sicknesses.

In ministering to people, we have seen many unexplainable diseases and sicknesses simply disappear when generational sins, curses and iniquities are dealt with.

Some may argue that Jesus became a curse for us and set us free from all curses. That's only a partial truth, just as not everyone is saved or born again even though Jesus died for the sin of the whole world.

Application is always required to receive the benefits of the cross. The purpose of mentioning this issue, is to make you aware of this area of hindrances to healing which is more prevalent than many realize. Sadly, much of the church doesn't have much understanding in this area, nor do they know how to effectively deal with it. It would take another book to reveal all that's involved and how to be set free. Although there are deliverance ministries which can be somewhat effective, they most often never deal with the root of the problems, which results in only partial or short lasting freedom.

What I recommend is a ministry such as "Restoring The Foundations" (RTF), or similar ministry that uses an integrated approach. Although a simplified explanation, RTF deals with four main areas which include: sins of the fathers or generational sins, ungodly beliefs, soul or heart wounds, and deliverance. Although my wife and I do RTF ministry, it's only one facet of our ministry, therefore because of time limitations, we confine it to pastors and leaders. My suggestion is to go on line for more information about "Restoring The Foundations," what it involves, and how to locate RTF ministers who may be in your area.

ESSENTIAL ELEMENTS WHEN PRAYING FOR OTHERS

The theme and the thread that runs from Genesis to Revelation isn't only our greatest need, but also the area in which we have the most difficulty in receiving and giving to others. **Love!** There is no other way to say this. Love, not your faith is the main substance that needs to flow from you to the ones you are praying for. You can pray without faith and your love and compassion for them will empower their own faith to rise up and they will be healed. The Bible says that out of love and compassion Jesus healed and set people free. Fourteen times in the Gospels, it says Jesus was moved with compassion for people. And compassion can only flow out of love. It's impossible to have genuine compassion if we don't have love. And it's impossible to have love without compassion coming out of that love.

Love must be the motivation to pray for people. I have observed too many, even though they see some success, are ministering out of duty or pride of putting another notch in their gun belt. It's easy to talk love, but until we understand how much God loves the person standing before us, our love and compassion for them can often come short and we end up mechanically praying and short circuiting the effectiveness of our prayers.

We are spirit beings and the spirit of the person we are praying for will know if we're praying out of love and compassion. Physically they may not know, but their heart and spirit will know. Obviously we're to see the person through God's eyes, but our love for them is tied directly to the degree we believe God loves us and how He sees us. As we grow in truly knowing God's love and compassion for us, we will discover that our love and compassion for others will also grow, and so too will the effectiveness of our prayers. God can and does move at times with mighty healings and miracles in spite of our lack of faith or love. But, to consistently see healing and miracles manifest we must make a lifestyle of living and basking in His love so it oozes out of us and into others.

Second or parallel to love we must possess faith and belief that God will heal the person in front of us. Not only that He'll heal someone's headache or backache, but that He will also heal the blind or the person in a wheelchair when we pray. We must come to a deep heart belief that the name of Jesus is above every name, which includes the name of cancer, blindness, diabetes, and other diseases that in the natural seem impossible. The real heart of our problem many times is that we subconsciously believe satan is greater than God.

A big tactic the devil often uses is to convince us that we have to muster up the power to heal the person, and that it's all up to us. We must come to true heart knowledge that God is the One who heals, but He has chosen to work through us.

The other essential when praying for

others is that the receiver's faith and belief plays a vital part in their healing. The Bible says that Jesus could do no mighty works in His own home town, so He set about to fix their inability to receive healing.

There will be times when you sense there is something hindering their faith, and they aren't in a position to be healed when you pray. If we pray when we're convinced they won't receive, that is time to stop and ask Holy Spirit for direction and how to proceed. Sometimes all it takes is encouragement that God truly loves them and that they will be healed when you pray. Just pause and listen to Holy Spirit for discernment. It may be an issue of unforgiveness, unworthiness, a demon or a combination of demonic and another issue.

It's never permissible to blame them or lay guilt on them for any lack of faith or issues of sin they may have. It's plain to see Jesus healed many who had sin in their lives, and I am sure in the multitudes, there were many who had no faith, but were healed by the faith of Jesus. Jesus never condemned or made them feel guilty as He prayed for. There's also never any room for you to feel guilty or condemned if the person isn't healed after you pray.

Our position is always to release the love and compassion of Jesus into them and to also receive it for ourselves. Whether there is instant manifestation or not, both the one praying and the one receiving prayer should leave feeling they are unconditionally and fervently loved by Jesus.

AN OPPORTUNITY TO
RECEIVE YOUR HEALING

I would like to close by having you pray this very simple prayer over yourself. Consider it your opportunity to receive your healing. In preparation, find a quiet place where you can silence your mind and spirit and invite the presence of Jesus. Whether you can sense His presence or not, you can be sure that He is there in your midst through Holy Spirit.

"God has said, "Never will I leave you; never will I forsake you." (Hebrews 13:5) NIV

Then simply believe for your miracle as you speak the following prayer out loud. In simple faith, receive Jesus as your healer, just as you received Him as your Savior. Receiving your healing is really that simple. *Jesus, I receive You as my healer and receive my healing that You paid for on the cross. In Your name, I command _____ (name the issue) to leave me and never return. In the*

name of Jesus, I command _____
(name the demonic spirits such as cancer, diabetes, pain) *to leave me and go to Jesus for reassignment. In the name of Jesus, I command*_____ (name the issue) *to be healed and all symptoms to leave and never return. I declare total healing has come to me and that I will live a long and prosperous life, totally free of disease, sickness and pain all the days of my life, and I will experience the goodness, favor and love of Jesus and my Father God, and the love of Holy Spirit all the days of my life. Amen!*

APENDIX

What follows are prayers and work sheets to address areas that can hinder the reception of healing. Included is a prayer to help you connect with God while taking communion, a short prayer of your identity and value to God, and a personalized prayer of Psalm 91. There is also a healing prayer for you to declare over yourself on a daily basis.

Upon contacting us we would be pleased to provide you with prayers tailored to deal with specific subjects or areas, such as witchcraft, Freemasonry, Occult, etcetera.

HEALING HEART WORKSHEET

Honestly facing our fears, angers, hatreds, resentments, judgments, hidden messages, and false labels, and then choosing to forgive those who have hurt us, relieves us of the need to set things straight or get even, and most important, gives us a life of freedom. It gives us the opportunity to break, nullify, and come out of agreement with curses, judgments, hidden messages and ungodly labels, which we have received from others, along with any judgments we may have placed upon them.

Circle each person who has wounded you, have hidden fear of, or have resentment, anger, hatred, bitterness, or unforgiveness towards. Then on a sheet of paper answer the questions listed. Before you begin, please read the short prayer below to invite Jesus and Holy Spirit into your healing session. Following this prayer is a short recap from the forgiveness section to help direct you in forgiveness and dealing with the painful emotions as you work through the worksheet.

Jesus, I ask You and Holy Spirit to please come to me in this time. I open the door for You and give you free access into my heart and into all my wounds and broken places, to lead me into wholeness and healing. I ask You to help me hear Your voice. Please don't let any other voice but Your's to speak Jesus. Lord Jesus, I belong to You alone and choose to give all I am in this process, my body, my soul and my spirit. Jesus, I trust You and Holy Spirit, and submit to Your authority so You can set me free.

WORKSHEET

Mother   Father   Sister   Brother
Grandparent   Spouse   Uncle   Aunt
Boyfriend   Girlfriend   Friend   Child
God   Spiritual Authority   Teacher   Others
Authority-Figures   Employer   Employee

Answer the questions in as much depth as possible. I have negative feeling against..........................
What did they do to me or what did they withhold that I needed from them? (the words or acts) How did they make me feel? (dirty, shameful, ugly, worthless, unwanted, etc).

What negative message did they send that I believe about myself? (I am a shameful person, I am unwanted, I am a failure, I am a liar, I am untrustworthy, etc.)

How have their words or actions affected my life? (I don't trust God or others, I am a cold person, I am fearful, I can't please anyone, God is never pleased with me, etc.)

PRAYERS TO REMOVE JUDGMENTS, WORD CURSES, UNGODLY EXPECTATIONS, NEGATIVE LABELS

Father, in the name of Jesus, I forgive _____ for what they did to me, for how their words and actions made me feel, and for the terrible effects it has had on my life. (name the actions, feelings, and the negative effects on your life).

In the name of Jesus I forgive. _____ for the negative message they sent me about my image or value, and for negative label/s they placed on me. (name the negative message/s and label/s unworthy, ugly, unwanted. _____

In the name of Jesus, I forgive _____ for any curses spoken over me, and for all the ungodly expectations placed upon me.

In Jesus' name, I forgive _____
for all judgments they made about me.

(These need to broke off, even if all the judgments, messages, expectations and labels are accurate and true, otherwise we will be imprisoned to live up to and according to them. The cycle needs to be broken).

In the name of Jesus, I come out of agreement with all the judgments, ungodly expectations, word curses and negative labels, placed on and against me by_____. I rebuke them and curse the very root of them, and command any demonic spirits assigned to keep them in place to be loosed and go to Jesus for reassignment.

When people wound us, we in turn end up judging them, release curses over them, place ungodly expectations on them and place labels on them, besides holding resentment, bitterness, hatred and unforgiveness etc. towards them. Luke 6:37-38 reveals that what we hold over them will return to us, multiplied many times and deposited in our hearts. Jesus said out of the abundance of the heart we will speak and will act. Therefore, after we have forgiven them for how they wounded us, it's very important to repent of our sinful responses towards them, by speaking the following prayer.

In the name of Jesus, I repent for all my negative responses against _____, and of all my judgments, ungodly expectations, word curses, and negative labels that I have place on and against _____.
Father, I receive Your forgiveness and forgive myself. Therefore, in the name of Jesus, I come out of agreement with all the judgments, ungodly expectations, word curses and negative labels that I have placed on and against _____. I rebuke them and curse the very root of them and command any demonic spirits assigned to keep them in place to be loosed and go to Jesus for reassignment.

PERSONAL APPLICATION

Picture the person in a prison cell. After asking Jesus for the key, unlock the door and take the person by the hand and lead them out of prison. Then look them in the eye and tell them exactly how they wounded you, including how it made you feel and how it damaged and affected your life. If you need to forgive your dad, you would first say something like, "dad, thank you for bringing me into the world, for providing food, clothing and a roof over my head," but then go on to tell him exactly how he wounded you, along with the feelings and lasting affects his actions had on your life.

For example, "Dad, you wounded me deeply, when you................ but through the power of Jesus, I am forgiving you and releasing you from all of my judgment."

Invite Jesus into the painful memories and situations. As you experience the emotions and pain, this is the time to hand the pain, trauma and memories to Jesus and picture what He does with them. Ask Him to heal all the wounds and brokenness in your heart.

Then take the person by the hand and lead them to Father God.

"Father this person has hurt me terribly and to be truthful, I have wanted to see them punished for what they did to me. But, I have forgiven and released them from all my anger and resentment. I no longer want to punish them and no longer want You to punish them for me. What I am asking is for You to set them in Your lap and put Your arms around them, and treat them like I wanted them to treat me. I am asking you to forgive and love them in the same way that I want You to forgive and love me."

Don't rush through this process. You don't want to short circuit what Jesus through Holy Spirit desires, and needs to do in order to bring healing and freedom in your life.

SPIRIT, SOUL AND BODY
TIES, ATTACHMENTS
AND TRANSFERS

Any time we spend time with someone, attachments, ties or transfers can take place in our spirits, souls and bodies. The depth or degree of transfer and connection is determined by the depth of relationship, and to the degree our souls were opened up to the other person. Ties can go both ways or one way, as when a baby is in a woman's womb. When a baby is in the womb, drugs, alcohol, negative emotional issues can transfer to the baby from the mother along with ties and attachments that will affect the baby all her or his life if not broken. Ties, attachments and transfers are taking place in every relationship. The good news is that we can deal with and control any ties coming upon us.

It is important to sever all the ties,

attachments and transfers to remove their negative effects and control over your life. Ties need to be broken if for example you had multiple relationships which may or may not have included sex, and then later married, you are bringing those persons into your married relationship. Every time you are being intimate with your spouse, you are also having your previous partners in bed with you through these ties and your marriage will be negatively affected. The same holds true if you were previously married, the ties need to be broken with your previous spouse, no matter if it was a great marriage or a bad one.

Breaking these ties can include more than the people and the incidents. In the case of a major trauma such as rape, besides naming the person/s involved and what happened, it's best to also include the location, sights, sounds, smells, and emotions you felt. Ties may need to be broken with parents, spouse, aunts, uncles, siblings, children, grandparents, sexual partners, (homosexual partners), authority figures, both secular & religious, ungodly prophecies and words, significant people in your life, organizations, clubs, false beliefs and religions, organizations and companies, buildings and land, people you idolized, blood pacts, ungodly vows, suicide, occult and witchcraft, both the people, practice and beliefs, drugs, sights, sounds, smells, places, words, beliefs, negative emotions such as fear, anger, etc. (idea is to name and break all ungodly connections to set us free from all that was harmful and negative in our lives).

Before proceeding with the prayer of breaking ties, please repent of any sin involved. Example: Repent and name each person you have had sex outside of marriage with, and receive God's forgiveness, and also forgive yourself for your part in the sin. Break ties with each person separately. If you can't remember names, just picture the person. It's best to deal with each person and incident separately.

Father, in the name of Jesus, I come to You and repent on behalf of myself and on behalf of everyone who played a part in establishing spirit, soul and body ties, connections or attachments that have had a negative impact on my life and on the life of others. I forgive myself and all those who have had a part in establishing these ties and connections.

In the name of Jesus, I sever and break all spirit, body and soul ties, transfers and attachments with_____. When finished with your list, pray the following:

In the name of Jesus, I not only sever and break all spirit, soul and body ties, attachments, and transfers, but I also send back to them everything that belongs to them that has tried to cling to me. And I take back everything that belongs to me washed in the blood of Jesus.

Father, in the name of Jesus Christ, I ask You to shut down all lines of communications in all dimensions of time and space that would keep these spirit, soul and body ties, attachments and transfers in place. I cancel and come out of agreement with any demonic entities assigned to keep these ties and connections in place. And, in the name of Jesus Christ, I command you to leave me now and go to Jesus for reassignment.

Heavenly Father, thank You for hearing my prayers, and for turning what the enemy meant for evil into Your blessings and favor upon my life. Amen!

HEALING DECLARATION

I encourage you to pray the following healing declaration our loud. It would be good to speak this prayer when you awake and also before you go to sleep. To achieve even more benefit, if you have the means, is to record the entire prayer, and then play it throughout the day and even when you are asleep. It's a proven fact that we trust our own voice above that of others.

Deuteronomy 28:61, says pain, all sickness, disease, infirmities and _____(name your issues) are a curse from not keeping the law.

But Galatians 3:13, says Christ has redeemed me from the curse of not keeping the Law. Therefore, I no longer have any pain, infirmities, diseases, sicknesses or_____, (name your issues).

I have the right to healing and freedom

from pain, sickness and disease. In the Name of Jesus, I exercise my rights and authority and command all pain, sickness, diseased and _____ to go!

Isaiah 53:4 & Matthew 8:17 says Jesus Himself, took pains, diseases, infirmities, and sicknesses, including _____ off of me and bore them on the cross. What He took off of me and bore, I don't need to bear! Therefore, since He bore all my pains, diseases, infirmities, sicknesses, including _____, I'm healed and free from them! I believe it in my heart and say it with my mouth. I am healed and well, therefore I can do the things that I couldn't do before.

Psalms 103:3-5 says, You continuously forgive all my sins and continuously heal all my diseases, and continuously redeem my life from the pit. You keep satisfying me with good things, and keep renewing my youth like the eagle's. I stay in faith and agreement with God.

1 Peter 2:21 says, by the stripes of Jesus I was healed, therefore I am presently healed. I agree with His Word that says I am already healed. God said it, I believe it, and that settles it!

I base my faith on what God says in His Word, not on what I see, hear, or feel. I'm not moved by what I see or feel. I'm moved only by what I believe! I don't care what the symptoms are. I believe that according to the Word of God that I'm healed.

In the face of symptoms, in the face of pain, in the face of that which is a lie, I believe and speak the truth because the Word of God is truth and His Word always works. God is known by His Word. He is everything the Word says He is, and He will do everything His Word says He will do. God and His Word are one.

In Isaiah 55:11, God said, I send out My word and it always produces fruit. It will accomplish all I want it to and it will succeed everywhere I send it. Therefore, I will see the results I want as I believe and line my words up with God's Word.

Psalms 107:20 says, God sent His Word and healed them. Since He didn't take His word back, it's still sent and has healed me. Therefore I no longer have pain, sickness, infirmities or any other disease.

I'm going to totally recover because Mark 16:18 says, they shall lay hands on the sick, and they shall recover.

I keep the switch of faith turned on. As I go about my day, the healing power of God is working in my body to bring healing and a cure. Every day I get better and better. Every day the healing power of God is working in my body. Every day I am able to do more and more.

Jesus, just as I accepted You as my Savior for life, I accept You as my Healer for life, therefore I no longer have to live with pain, diseases, infirmities or sicknesses.

I base my faith on what I know from God's Word, not on human reasoning or understanding. I operate out of my spirit, not out of my head.

Philippians 2:13 says God is working in me both to will and to do of His good pleasure. It's God's good pleasure for me to be healed and made whole, because healing is His will for my life.

God's Word always works, and His Word abides in me. I put my faith in His Word, and because I ask according to His will for healing, it shall be done unto me.

Jesus, as I walk close to You in faith, Your healing power drives out all pain, sickness and disease from my body.

I can't rely on another person's faith to get things done in my own life. I must believe God's Word in my own heart and speak His Word out of my own mouth.

I'm so glad I don't have to wait for a sovereign move of God. I can believe what the Bible says. And according to First Peter 2:24, I have already been healed.

Because I have a free will, I can choose to follow God and enjoy all of His many benefits or go against Him and suffer.

Holy Spirit, show me anything that isn't in line with God's will or desire, and anything that's preventing me from receiving a full manifestation of healing.

Jesus, as I walk close to You, I will see my complete healing manifested. I call those things that are not yet manifested in the natural as though they already exist. In the face of sickness, I see and call my body healed and well, and see myself living life to the fullest.

I don't base my faith on what I see or feel or on what other people say or think. I base my faith on God's word. I hear with the ears of faith, see with the eyes of faith and only speak the Words of faith. I command every part of my body to function as it was designed to function.

I refuse to let doubt rob me of the blessings of God. I shut the door on doubt. I choose instead to believe and act on what God's Word says. I believe what God says before I ever see anything in the natural. I act on God's Word, and as I do, I see miracles happen in my life. I don't act presumptuously or foolishly by just giving mental ascent to God's Word, but let it get down on the inside of me so I can act in true faith. And when I do, I get results.

I don't have to try and get faith. I already have faith. I simply act on what God says in His Word and believe by the stripes of Jesus that I am already healed and made whole.

I'm not moved by what I see or by what I feel. I'm moved only by what I believe with my heart. I listen to my heart, not to my physical senses. I believe I am healed no matter what my physical senses tell me.

If I'm worried or anxious, then I'm not believing that God will meet every need in my life. As I trust His Word that I'm healed, rest will come in my spirit.

Jesus in me is greater than sickness and disease, and He always causes me to triumph in Him. The same spirit that raised Jesus from the dead lives in me and gives life to my physical body.

I shall live and not die and declare the glory of the Lord. I give God's Word first place in my life and listen to what He says, rather than the words of people. I know God is with me and in me, so I don't have to fear. God will help and strengthen me and uphold me with His right hand.

I guard my mouth and only speak what lines up with God's Word. In my heart I believe I'm healed and well, so I speak it out of my mouth. I know that death and life are in the power of my tongue. I line my words up with what God says about me. I believe I'm healed, so I constantly speak words of health and healing out of my mouth.

I take heed to the Word of God and receive it with an open mind and heart. I meditate on the Word and speak forth out of my heart that I am healed. I walk by faith in God's Word, rather than what I can see with my physical eyes.

I believe I am who God says I am and that I can do what God says I can do. I brag about who I am in Christ and what God has done for me. God has given me all things that pertain to life and godliness. I speak out what belongs to me in Christ. I thank God for all of His many blessings!

If my speaking is wrong, it's because my believing is wrong. If my believing is wrong, it's because my thinking is wrong. I choose to think God's thoughts. I search the Word of God to find out what God says about me and my situation. Then I apply God's Word to my life. I think on it, believe it, and speak it out of my mouth! My confession is in line with what God said.

Confession is declaring what I believe is true, testifying to something I know in my heart, and witnessing to a truth I have embraced. I glorify God with a right confession and bring about the devil's defeat in every difficult situation in my life.

I keep the door closed on the devil and I don't allow him into any part of my life. I am careful to only speak words that bring glory and honor to God. I don't talk fear because God hasn't given me a spirit of fear, but the spirit of power, love and a sound mind. As I declare that I have a spirit of power, love and a sound mind it will become a reality in my life.

God anointed Jesus. And then Jesus did good things with that anointing. God anointed me with power and I will do good things with the anointing!

The power of God is greater than the power

of the devil and greater than pain, sickness or disease, therefore God's power drives out all pain, sickness and disease in my body.

There's nothing too difficult for God. No matter how long it has been or how impossible it may seem, God can turn any situation or condition around! I am healed, not by my effort or by my power, but by God's Spirit. The anointing of God heals me.

God is bigger than a doctor's report or any negative report. I know the healing power of God works, so I cooperate with His power in my life and I am able to do what I couldn't do before!

The healing power of God is working in my body at this very instant to bring healing and a cure. From the moment the healing power of God goes into my body, I begin to heal. And each day, no matter what it looks or feels like, I am getting better and better, and will see the full manifestation of my healing.

Faith and God's power are an unbeatable combination! I mix my faith with His power to receive total healing. Pain, infirmities, sickness and disease are no match for God. I overcome because greater is He who is in me than he who is in the world! The Greater One is in me. He is greater than any pain, infirmity, sickness or disease. He is greater than distress, anxiety or fear. He is greater than the enemy. He is greater than any test, trial, or anything I might face!

The Healer is in me, and is working in my body to bring forth healing and health. I've claimed healing and health, therefore pain, infirmity, sickness and disease, you have to go!

God wants me well. It's the will of God for me to be healthy and to live the full length of my life down here on earth without sickness, infirmity, pain, or disease. That's the will of God! I accept His will today. I believe I receive healing from the top of my head to the soles of my feet. It's easy to receive healing.

God responds to faith because faith pleases God. Faith puts God's power to work. When my faith is coupled with the power of God, there is a supernatural explosion that meets my every need!

I don't have to have a special kind of faith to receive healing. I can use the same faith that saved me. Because my disease and sickness were laid upon Jesus, I declare I healed and free. I accept as truth that Jesus bore my pain, infirmity, disease, and sickness, including _____, therefore I declare I have been healed and made whole.

I speak the Word of God. I speak faith-filled, life-filled words that change the circumstances around me. I refuse to speak doubt and unbelief. I refuse to give up; I refuse to quit. I know that health and healing belong to me.

As I meditate on and declare the promises of God, I will see the full manifestation in my body. I see every symptom leaving and see myself well, living a long pain free, healthy life.

As a child of God, I am part of the body of Jesus, and as His representative, the authority of His name belongs to me. I am fully authorized to use the Name of Jesus along with the authority that He has given me in His Name to be healed, and to set myself and others free.

Therefore I command all symptoms of pain, infirmities, sicknesses and diseases to leave me now in the name of Jesus Christ. And, I command any demonic spirits assigned to keep any symptoms in place to be loosed from me and go to Jesus for reassignment. Thank You Jesus! Amen and Amen.

SELF WORTH PRAYER

Jesus, thank You for creating me in such a wonderful way. Your Word says I was not only fine crafted or woven like beautiful tapestry in my mother's womb, but that You only have precious thoughts about me. Which mean that I am your precious son/daughter. (Psalm 139:13, 17)

Father, I am so thankful that it was Your idea to bring me into Your family as Your son/daughter. It is so good to know I am wanted and am so valued by You. (John 1:12)

Father, I am so grateful that You valued me so highly and truly wanted me as Your son/daughter, so much so that You paid for my redemption by sending Your Son to be crucified on my behalf. Jesus, You have promised to supply all my needs according to Your riches in glory. Thank Your that I can be at peace knowing You will take care of all my needs. (Philippians 4:19)

Father, thank You that because Jesus died and set me free from sin and from being Your enemy in my mind and in my actions, that You now see me as holy, blameless and above reproach. (Colossians 1:19-23)

Holy Spirit, I ask You to never allow me to forget how much I am loved and valued by the Godhead. Please help me to learn how to receive love from the Father, so I may then be able to give love and receive love from others.

Holy Spirit, Please alert me anytime I begin to listen or come into agreement with the lies from the enemy of my soul. And, also help me to no longer listen to any lies from my formative years that have wounded me and cause me to form wrong beliefs about myself and You.

Holy Spirit, I surrender every part of my being, and give You permission to work in my life until I am formed into the image of Jesus.

PRAYER FOR TAKING DAILY COMMUNION

I encourage you to take daily communion, as it truly is the meal that heals. Jesus never meant it to be a ritual which results in very little connection with Jesus and His sacrifice. I personally try to take communion at least once per day first thing in the morning and often when possible at night before bed.

Try not to rush through this prayer, but meditate on the aspects of what Jesus did for us. This is not meant to be a ritual prayer to use on a continual basis, but rather to help jumpstart you on going deeper with connecting and identifying with the suffering of Jesus and what He accomplished on the cross for you. Your own heartfelt prayer is what will bring you into communion with Jesus and what He did for you on the cross.

Jesus, I come to You just as I am with all of my strengths and all my weaknesses, all my failures and imperfections, and all of my needs.

Jesus, my heart is overwhelmed by Your love for me, which You demonstrated when You were crucified on my behalf. As much as possible, I want to identify with You and Your suffering for me as I try to imagine each facet of your crucifixion.

Thank You for how You suffered on my behalf in the Garden, as You were abandoned by Your disciples, as You were shamed, reviled and spit upon, as You were beaten with fists and rods, as the crown of thorns was jammed and beat down with rods, as You were scourged tearing Your flesh from Your body, and as You were mocked when You were crucified unjustly in my place.

Jesus, I don't want Your suffering to be wasted or be in vain, therefore in faith, as I prophetically eat of Your body, I receive all the healing You paid for into every area of my soul, into every area of my body, and into every area of my life.

Thank You for shedding Your blood to set me free from the curse and penalty of my sin and iniquity.

Jesus, as I prophetically drink the cup of Your blood, I receive Your total forgiveness and total washing away of all my sins and iniquities through Your shed blood. I receive the cleansing power of Your blood to wash over every area of my soul, over my will, over my conscience, over my imagination, over my memories, over my desires, over my motives, over my speaking, over my actions, and over my way of thinking.

Jesus, thank You for sealing me into Your new covenant and giving me new life.

PERSONALIZED DAILY PRAYER OF PSALM 91

Because I dwell in the secret place of the Most High, I find rest under the shadow of the Almighty. You are the eternal Jehovah God, and You alone are my refuge, my place of safety and my mighty God, and I will always trust in You.

Surely You will deliver me from every trap of the enemy, from every calamity, every destruction, every sickness and every disease. You cover me with Your feathers, and under Your wings I find shelter.

Because Your truth is my armor and protection, I'm not afraid of any terror by night, any daytime attacks, or any disease that walks in darkness, or any disaster that comes day or night. A thousand may fall at my side and ten thousand at my right hand, but it won't come near me. Only with my eyes will I look and see the reward of the wicked.

Lord, because I have made You my refuge and my dwelling place, no evil will befall or conquer me, nor shall any disease or plague come near me or my house; For You shall give Your angels charge over me to protect me everywhere I go. They hold me so securely in their hands that I won't even stub my foot against a stone.

I will trample upon all the destructive powers of the spirit world, including loud and venomous demonic voices, and I will crush the serpent under my feet.

Lord God, because I have set my love upon You, I am confident You will always deliver me. You will set me on high, because I have known Your Name.

When I call upon You, You will answer me quickly. You will be with me in times of trouble and will not only deliver and honor me, but You will satisfy me with long life as I live each day experiencing Your wonderful salvation.

ABOUT THE AUTHOR

John Mark Volkots, a former pastor, along with his wife Ramona, are itinerant ministers with hearts to bring the Father's love to the nations, through teaching, preaching, and Father Heart Encounter/ Schools. Their desire is to see people discover and live out of their true Godly identity, and to receive a revelation of a God Who dearly loves His children. They also provide personal ministry to leaders, ministers and others who need healing of wounded hearts.

For more information on the author and their ministry, please visit: healing4thenations.net.

For questions, feedback or other inquires Email at: jmvolkots@gmail.com

It would also be appreciated if you would leave a review on Amazon.

OTHER BOOKS BY THE AUTHOR AVAILABLE IN PAPERBACK AND ON KINDLE

A JOURNEY INTO THE HEART OF GOD
The Bible was meant to be a pathway into a deep relationship with our creator. But our modern life is a whirlwind, overwhelming us with cell phones, movies, social media, and much noise, choking out quality time with the lord. Many don't have a deep relationship with God, however it should be normal for all believers. This book is meant to provide a way into a deep relationship with God in the midst of this complex, busy, and noisy world. Your relationship with God can be all that you desire, and your view of yourself, and of the Lord will be forever changed. I invite you to begin your own personal journey into the heart of God.

7 KEYS TO EXPERIENCE KINGDOM LIFE

Nearly every Christian I have met has desired to live a fulfilled, joyful and victorious life, yet it seems that very few ever achieve that goal on a daily basis. It is not that they haven't wanted it, but far too many struggle to attain it. Yet the Bible describes it as the normal life for the early church. Paul said, "the Kingdom of God is not eating and drinking, but righteous, peace and joy." Jesus said, "seek the Kingdom of God and all these things shall be added to you. Do not fear little flock, for it is your Father's good pleasure to give you the Kingdom." He also said, "I will give you the keys to the Kingdom." 7 KEYS TO EXPERIENCE KINGDOM LIFE will reveal how you can discover heart attitudes that will allow you to throw off the chains, strongholds and darkness that have been holding you back from living a victorious Kingdom life on a daily basis.

A to Z CHRISTIAN DREAM SYMBOL DICTIONARY Contains the meanings of over 2400 symbols to assist and train you in unlocking the mysteries of your dreams and the dreams of others. Understanding the meaning of dream symbols can help you discover what your dream means, and far more important can help you discover the message it contains for your life.

WHAT A CRAZY LIFE One man's journey in life, and how stupid, brilliance and a great imagination can live together in one person Guaranteed to make you laugh, but far more important is that you will discover how God takes a person with normal weaknesses, and uses all things that are good along with the not so good things, and works them for His and our good. Even more important however, is that as You read, will also discover the love and favor that God wants to bestow on all of us.

RECLAIMING THE KINGDOM OF GOD Jesus died so we could have total victory over the devil and sin. Yet, far too many aren't experiencing that victory! Many of God's people often suffer from the same depression, suppression and oppression as non-Christians. In the modern church, fornication, adultery, divorce, greed, anger, bitterness, and other sins nearly parallel those of the world. Many put on a religious disguise in church, but their daily lives are anything but victorious. Some are just empty shells hoping for the Lord's return to end their misery and take them to heaven. The sad part is that they believe what they have is the normal Christian life. The truth is that they are settling for a counterfeit religious form of Christianity! RECLAIMING THE KINGDOM OF GOD is designed to help you rediscover what the early church experienced. You can truly be free from the bondages of this world, and free to live what should be the normal joyful and victorious Christian life on a continual basis.